CONTENTS

INTRODUCTION

I've been fascinated by health and nutrition for over twenty years, beginning at age 19 when I became a competitive bodybuilder and I would eat an entire rack of ribs every day for a week leading up to a competition. In my mid-twenties (no longer bodybuilding), I became a vegan, primarily for ethical reasons, but I dove deeply into the available science and pro-vegan literature, and I believed veganism was the healthiest way to eat. I then delved deeply into raw food veganism. I became a trained raw vegan chef, blogger, and cookbook author. I was deeply committed to veganism and built a whole career around it.

Then one day, I realized that my toddler daughter was not thriving. This was despite my very serious commitment to providing her with what I believed was a nutritionally complete diet and spending a small fortune in the highest quality supplements available. The full story of my transition from vegan, to "reformed vegan," to elk-heart-eating, bloodthirsty carnivore is laid out briefly in this book, and in even more detail (for those who are interested) in one of my most highly trafficked blog posts of all time, as well as in an interview with Dave Asprey on his Bulletproof Radio podcast (for details, see Resources, Chapter 16).

The short version is that I've done a *complete, 180-degree reversal* from my plants-only diet days. I now eat almost zero plants, except for occasional, specific medicinal purposes (some plants have powerful pharmacological compounds). The reasons why, the potential benefits, and "how to" instructions for trying the carnivore diet for yourself are what this book is all about.

Here's what the book is not: I'm not trying to promote or advocate for the carnivore diet. My diet is a lifelong experiment and a work-in-progress. I have no idea if I'll still be eating this way in a year or decade from now.

Two things I know for sure:

1) I learned my lesson with veganism.

Early positive results don't necessarily indicate long-term success. Everybody is different, everyone's genome and circumstances are different, and YMMV ("your mileage may vary"). I will never be dogmatic again. I will try to keep my cognitive biases in check... and confirmation bias is a powerful beast. It's best to approach diet and nutrition with an open mind, even if that means periodically questioning things you're "certain" about. Even if you were right, your body changes with age.

2) The current state of nutrition science *ABSOLUTELY SUCKS*.

The scientists do their best with their limited tools and inadequate funding, but the simple truth is that due to financial, time, ethical, and practical constraints, we have virtually zero well-designed, long-term, experimental studies with significantly large groups to suss out what's best for human health, fitness, and longevity.

Instead of good science, we have a maddening mishmash of n=10, six-month microstudies and thousands of flawed, often contradictory, correlational studies that do their best to determine what the hell is actually going on inside of us. It's a total mess. (No one is to blame; it's just a really difficult problem and there are no financial incentives for anyone to spend moon-shot amounts of money to solve it today.)

At some point in the distant future, we'll have the data and sensor technology to fully map all of the trillions of interconnected chemical pathways in the human body, a complete understanding of epigenetics, and we'll have computers and AI algorithms powerful enough to accurately model human physiology, down to the molecular level. In that future, we'll be able to sequence your DNA and monitor your blood in real-time and tell you exactly what, and how much, to eat for any given goal. And it will usually be correct.

Until then... you're on your own. You are the scientist with total, unfettered access to "population = you" and you get to experiment every day with your own body. Find out what works and doesn't work best for you. Actually, you're not on your own. You have lively online communities of people sharing their stories and results. It's not great data, but they are data points comprising lots of crowd-sourced trial and error. And most of all, plenty of ideas and encouragement for your own experimentation. If you're new to the world of carnivory, this book can serve as an introduction to that community and a starting point for your own scientific journey of discovery and personal success.

Disclaimer – Read This, It's Important

I'm not a doctor, nurse, pharmacist, nutritionist, or scientist. (I'm also not a midwife, financial advisor, spiritual guru, or astronaut.) This book is not intended to give medical advice. This book is not intended to tell you how you should eat or what you should do.

The information in this book is strictly to share my experiences from going on a carnivore diet and the anecdotal data I've collected in researching it for myself. You should always seek the guidance of a doctor, preferably one knowledgeable about various diets and natural living, before making any major lifestyle changes like diet and fitness.

I wish there had been a book like this when I started. That's why I wrote it. My goal is to provoke thought about a carnivore diet and share tips for doing it, as well as resources that you can explore further. Like I said about my lesson from veganism, I do not aim to be dogmatic about the carnivore diet. I do not have all the answers, and I hope you approach this book with an open mind.

I'm also not suggesting that everyone subscribe to a strict, meat-only diet. I do not think there is enough evidence to support that yet. Until a lot more (and better) studies are done, it's up to you to figure out what makes you feel best. Perhaps you'll thrive on a strict, meat-only diet, or perhaps you're wired to function best with only a "meat-heavy" diet, or not even that. Either way, the following pages will give you some insight on why I started eating a carnivore diet, how I did it, tips for transitioning, and (of course) recipes to get you started.

CHAPTER 1: WHAT IS THE CARNIVORE DIET?

Eating a carnivore diet is exactly what you would think:

- You eat animal products (and by-products).
- You do not eat plants (vegetables, nuts, seeds, grains, legumes, fruits).

The carnivore diet is also known as a "zero-carb" diet, or "all-meat" diet, although zero carb is a bit misleading as olive oil is a zero-carb plant, and therefore, not on a carnivore diet. Also, eggs have a trace amount of carbohydrate. Full-fat dairy, such as cheese and whipping cream, also have trace amounts of carbohydrate. Therefore, when you eat a so-called "zero-carb" diet, it could have a trace amount of carbohydrate, depending on the animal foods you eat.

Still, some people on a carnivore diet consider these technicalities to be splitting hairs and they call it a zero-carb diet because it has essentially no carbs.

What Can I Eat on a Carnivore Diet?

There are a few ways to approach the carnivore diet.

You might think, "How is that? Seems pretty simple… eat animals and don't eat plants. Got it." True, that is the diet in its most basic form. But from there, you've got a lot of options.

A carnivore diet can include any of the following foods:

- Beef
- Buffalo
- Chicken
- Eggs
- Duck
- Turkey
- Pork
- Fish
- Lamb/mutton
- Rabbit
- Venison/elk
- Goat
- Oyster, Crab, Lobster, Shrimp, Squid, Octopus
- Offal (liver, kidney, tongue, heart, etc)
- Insects

- Snake, alligator, frog legs
- Dairy (whole-fat choices are best: cheese, yogurt, milk, heavy cream, butter, and ghee)

That's a lot of choices. Furthermore, there are different ways to prepare these foods for a plethora of meat-heaven diversity. Roasted, stewed, grilled, steamed, seared, etc.

Two things worth noting:

1. Over time, it's common for carnivore dieters to gravitate to a beef-heavy diet. It happened to me, too. It's easy, delicious, and the desire for variety just starts to dwindle. I've read about carnivore dieters who eat only beef and drink only water. That's it. There are others who are even more specific in eating only ribeye steaks and drinking water.

2. Many carnivore dieters avoid dairy or consume it only occasionally. If they do have dairy, it's always full-fat (cheese, butter, ghee, heavy cream).

Beef and Dairy

The reason many carnivore dieters eat mostly beef, especially fatty cuts, over other animal products, is because it's nutrient dense and extremely satisfying. The fatty part is absolutely key to high nutrition and satiety, so I never trim the fat and I eat it all.

Like the other carnivore dieters, I too migrated to preferring mostly beef after a while. At first, I wanted variety. I feared getting bored, so I consumed pork, chicken, fish, and dairy.

Over the course of two months eating carnivore, however, I noticed that I most desired beef, especially fatty ribeye steaks. Oh, how I loved the fat on those. Over time, I ate less pork, dairy, and chicken. They still made appearances, as does offal (for nutrition when my badassery is strong enough), but they weren't the norm for me.

As for dairy, the main reasons that many carnivores go without it is allergies, or just plain not feeling as optimal with dairy added. They might on occasion get cheese on a beef patty, but most days they go without dairy. My husband, on the other hand, loves cheese and thinks that eating a beef patty without cheese is a waste of a cow. He loves his breadless "cheeseburger" (just a 1/2-pound ground beef patty with melted cheese on it) and likes to say, "nobody ever wrote a song called *Hamburger in Paradise*."

I, too, have dairy on occasion, but not often. There are those times when I come home and haven't eaten in 7 hours, I'm hungry, and I still have to cook dinner. The perfect snack for me is an ounce or two of cheese. It totally takes the edge off of hunger until I cook up a proper pound of ground beef or steak.

Dairy was a smart choice for me when I was transitioning to the carnivore diet. It's tasty and satisfying.

Do People Need Vegetables?

There is a surprising lack of research on this. It's entirely possible that we don't. Many experts say that carbohydrates are not essential, whereas nobody says that protein and fats are not essential. Vitamins and minerals can be obtained from animal sources. That leaves the question of specific phytonutrients (plant compounds), and science has only just begun to ask the somewhat heretical question of whether these are necessary in the context of a diet with no plants.

What we do know is that there are people around the world and some civilizations through history who subsisted primarily on a diet very low in carbs. And for many cultures, there were times when carbohydrates were only available certain times of the year. So, it seems that there were people who survived for generations without eating carbohydrates every day.

But Aren't Veggies Good for Me?

It's not as simple as you'd think. Let's look at the beloved broccoli, for example.

According to Dr. Georgia Ede,

"Public health officials and nutrition experts love to sing the praises of the virtuous cruciferous vegetable family. How does sulforaphane kill tiny living creatures, and why should you care? … In research studies it has also been demonstrated that sulforaphane can kill healthy human cells and can cause cancerous changes in human cells. It may come as a surprise to you to learn that this sulforaphane is the very same broccoli ingredient that we are told is responsible for the health benefits of broccoli. Why do we only hear about broccoli's superhero side, and not its villainous dark side?

"… The belief that vegetables are good for us comes entirely from epidemiological studies, which are only capable of generating untested theories about food and health. Scientific experiments are then conducted to try to support those beliefs, and the truth is that these experiments yield very mixed results about how broccoli affects us."

Yes, people can derive nutrition from plants, but it's important to realize that some people are more sensitive to the compounds in plants than others. And, some people might not even realize it unless they try the carnivore diet, as an elimination diet, to find out.

So, if you are *super* sensitive to plants, you might feel best when you don't consume them so frequently, but, if you have some now and then (say once a week or every other week), it's not going to have any real detrimental effect on your health. It might be enjoyable even. For others, they have found that they can't have any plants without it causing them much discomfort.

For myself, I no longer see plants as a great source of nutrition. At least not for now. I'm still feeling healthy and fine without them. Admittedly, the human body can withstand a fair amount of bullshit for a while, so we'll have to wait and see.

Now I see plants more as medicine than food. That's an important role to play, but it doesn't mean I want to take medicine every day, especially if I don't have a specific condition I'm trying to heal.

If I were a sick person, I'd first be looking at how I feel without carbohydrates, because that could be a key. Then, if I needed, I'd consider adding some fruits or vegetables, extracts, herbs or spices for medicinal reasons. However, I'm aware that just because a study shows some isolated (and concentrated) compound from broccoli or turmeric, for instance, has a benefit doesn't mean if I start eating a bunch of broccoli or turmeric that I'll get those benefits.

For starters, I may not be getting the quantity of the compound that I would need for it to be effective. Second, there may be other compounds in the broccoli causing me harm in servings large enough to get the required dosage.

Carnivore Diet Sounds Weird. Is It Dangerous?

I know what people are wondering. It is weird? Is it dangerous?

It was weird to me, at first. Eating only meat runs contrary to conventional nutrition wisdom, such as "you need to eat a lot of vegetables, fiber, and grains.

But, consider this. According to Dr. Georgia Ede:

"As outrageous as this may sound, I find no scientific evidence that vegetables are essential components of the human diet, because I am not aware of a single study that compares a diet containing vegetables to a diet without vegetables."

And this:

"To the best of my knowledge, the world has yet to produce a civilization which has eaten a vegan diet from childhood through death, whereas there are numerous examples throughout recorded history of people from a variety of cultural, ethnic and geographical backgrounds who have lived on mainly-meat diets for decades, lifetimes, generations. To my mind, examples of real people eating mostly-meat diets for long periods of time gives us much more powerful information about meat and health than conventional scientific studies conducted over short periods of time in which one group of people eats a little more meat or a few extra servings of vegetables than another group of people."

The Inuit, Plains Indians, Mongolians, and Masai are only a few of the more well-known meat-heavy cultures (meaning they ate a "mostly meat" diet most of the time). For the North American Plains Indians, the bison was famously the "staff of life" since prehistoric times, and they lived primarily on this and other game animals.

These cultures also thrived. This means we do have information and accounts of meat-eating cultures *and* their good health. They had an absence of most of the diseases we suffer from in today's world that eats a lot of plants, especially grains. That made me curious. *What if people don't actually need to eat plants?* There's more to health than just food though. These people were not eating meat off the bone all day, hunched over a computer. They were very active – many of them were nomadic, following the game herds – meaning they got a lot of exercise. Their lives depended on plenty of walking or running. Diet is important for health and longevity, but it's not the only factor. It's one of many things in my toolkit.

Context is important when we speak of "plants." Remember, this is about the *whole* plant kingdom, not just fruits and vegetables. If someone is eating an omnivore diet of meat and grains, then substituting the grains with fruits and vegetables will absolutely offer better *nutrition*. But the question of whether we can get everything we need from meat – that is, whether we actually need *any* plants (grains, fruits, vegetables, etc.) instead of eating a totally carnivore diet… well… it defies conventional wisdom, but I'm currently not convinced that we need plants anymore. I suspect that it might be possible to get everything we need from animal products.

Highsteaks.com provides an entertaining article questioning whether you need veggies to be healthy. Here are a few of the highlights (though the <u>entire article</u> is worth a read).

- *Animal foods provide all the micronutrients a person needs.*
- *Animal products include some of the most nutrient-dense foods available. They're our best (and often only) source of vitamin A (retinol), DHA/EPA, and vitamin B12, as well as lesser-known nutrients like choline, creatine, and carnosine.*
- *There are plenty of nutrients we NEED in animal foods that can only be found in animal foods, but none in plants that are unavailable in animal foods.*
- *Plants have lots of nutrients, but they're not a "good" source, as they come with plenty of "anti-nutrients" which bind to the same receptors and reduce uptake by the body, or are destroyed by cooking, or are unavailable without certain fats.*
- *Eat veggies if you want – not because they're "healthy", but because they can be delicious… (And to keep Mom happy.)*

Is Eating a Carnivore Diet Dangerous?

To the best of my knowledge, based on a great deal of research, I don't believe that eating a carnivore diet is dangerous. While there is a lack of clinical research, I've come to this conclusion based on 1) the anthropological evidence (above), 2) other people's anecdotal success with the diet, and 3) based on my own experience with it so far.

Conversely, I consider processed foods and refined sugars as the dangerous foods, not meat. Eating lots of steaks doesn't scare me. I am eating this way because I simply feel better when I do, and I seem to be able to stay in great shape and maintain muscle mass with less exercise than I used to do when I was on an omnivore diet.

And as of now, I'm simply happier on a carnivore diet. I feel it every day, and it's undeniable. If drinking green smoothies every day made me feel great, I'd do that, but it doesn't.

What About Heart Disease? Aren't I Concerned About Cholesterol and Saturated Fat?

In a word, no.

For those who haven't heard, the theory stating that dietary cholesterol is linked to coronary heart disease has been largely disproved. This flawed theory was based on bad science that resulted in shifting the entire population toward a "low-fat" (i.e., high-carb) diet for thirty years, to deadly effect, with epidemic levels of obesity, diabetes, and more.

Unfortunately, old habits die hard and there are still lots of doctors (and, ahem, pharmaceutical companies), and purveyors of truly shitty food that either haven't gotten the memo or have some misaligned incentives to continue pushing carbs at the expense of much healthier fat.

To repeat my disclaimer from the introduction, I'm not a doctor, and I'm not recommending a carnivore diet to people. There are plenty of people (and many experts) who say without reservation that the carnivore diet is safe to try and you shouldn't be afraid. After all, a person can always just take it day by day. If you don't feel well, switch back, no harm done.

If you're still concerned, you could always visit your doctor before you begin this (or any) new diet to get bloodwork (a "lipid panel") to establish a baseline. Then repeat in three or six months to see how things have changed.

What About Vitamin C? What About Fiber? What About…

These are great questions. The experts advocating the carnivore diet address them directly. The short version is that metabolic chemistry and nutritional requirements are very different once you eliminate plants from your diet, and conventional observational studies don't apply because they haven't studied groups of carnivores.

For the long version, see Chapter 5, Frequently Asked Questions About the Carnivore Diet.

Carnivore Diet vs. Keto Diet

Supporting the idea that the carnivore diet is not dangerous is the fact that it's not very different from the already popular "keto" diets that many people have been doing for years (and used for certain medical therapies, such as treating epilepsy). A ketogenic diet is a diet high in fat, adequate in protein, and low enough in carbohydrates that it forces the body to shift its metabolism to burn fats. In addition to specific medical uses, keto diets are popular with athletes and fitness enthusiasts who seek a high-muscle, low-fat body composition… which is basically all of them except powerlifters and sumo wrestlers. Most people going to a carnivore diet don't do it with the aim at ketosis, but it's a potential side benefit.

It's Early Days Still, but the Results Look Promising

It's great to see other people catching on to the carnivore way of eating as they read about others having such success. There's been an upswing in the movement lately. These people are reporting that their health is thriving. In fact, for some, it's the only thing they *can* do to thrive. The carnivore diet could have a powerful impact for helping with many diseases.

The common experience is that someone hears about it and thinks it's insane. Then, they read a bit and think it might not be so crazy. Then, they try it and see how simple it is, cravings go away, they feel great, and they want to keep doing it.

Reported Benefits of the Carnivore Diet

Let's start with the commonly reported benefits of people eating a carnivore diet. Again, your mileage may vary. These results don't always happen with everyone. Diet, though it plays a huge role, is only one of many factors in determining health. That said, I personally find it exciting to see these testimonials from people after they started a carnivore diet!

- **Improved skin**, including clearing of skin tags, clearing of acne, eliminating eczema, and anti-aging effects seen on the skin as anti-inflammatory foods replace carbohydrates in the diet.

- **Carbohydrate cravings *finally* disappear.** This usually happens after going through a 1-3 week transition period if the person is coming from a carbohydrate-rich diet. For people coming from a keto diet, they are already more fat-adapted and carb cravings can be eliminated much faster. Once the cravings disappear, it sticks. Plop a piece of cake in front of one of these folks, and they have no problem passing on it. Desire just isn't there. In my case, I'd much rather have a ribeye.

- **Fat loss.** There are countless testimonials showing people losing weight on a carnivore diet. Want to spend thirty minutes getting really inspired? Visit MeatHeals.com and browse the before-and-after carnivore diet pictures. People lose weight and gain energy. It's effortless because they're satisfied on the diet (meat is, after all, delicious), and cravings are controlled or non-existent. On the flip side, some people can gain weight... in a good way. If a person comes to the diet with malnourishment, it's possible to gain some weight, maybe only temporarily, as the body rebuilds and changes from a carbohydrate-driven metabolism to a fat-adapted one. Some people therefore argue that the carnivore diet isn't a "weight-loss" diet, but rather, that it burns fat and promotes muscle growth, making it an overall "improved body composition" diet.

- **Increased testosterone in men.** According to a study in the *American Journal of Clinical Nutrition*, men who ate a 10-week diet high in fat, low in fiber, saw an increase in testosterone 13% higher than the low-fat, high-fiber group. Anecdotally, Ryan Munsey, a performance coach with a degree in food science and human nutrition (ryanmunsey.com), went carnivore for 35 days and ate 2-4 pounds of meat daily. His testosterone jumped from 495 ng/dL to 569.

- **Reduction of pain** and incidence of migraine headaches.

- **Reduced joint aches** and injuries with lowered inflammation.

- **Improvement in allergies** This applies to both food allergies (because of the eliminative nature of the carnivore diet and the healing that takes place) and seasonal allergies.

- **Increased libido**.

- **Simplicity.** It's a simple diet that is easy to start and quite effortless to maintain. There are no complicated recipes to follow and much less time is spent in the grocery store and kitchen.
- **Improved digestion** and less time in the bathroom trying to poop for long periods of time. Some people report dramatic improvements (life-changing) in their digestive disorders as a result of no longer eating irritating foods.
- **Improved sleep** with many reports of needing less sleep.
- **Improved cognition and focus.**
- **Strength gains and improved recovery time.** Athletes have experienced gains in strength and quicker recovery from protein and nutrient-rich foods like beef and a reduction in inflammatory foods.
- **Easier muscle maintenance.** Some people have reduced the intensiveness of workouts while eating carnivore, yet find they're able to maintain muscle and have great definition. (I've found personal joy in this one, as we travel abroad without access to a gym.)
- **Feeling better mentally, with dramatic mood improvement.** People report depression going away. They're empowered, and they feel happy and strong. Confidence in abundance as they experience high performance.

I'd highly recommend scouring the internet to read people's stories about going on a carnivore diet. It's really inspiring. In the Resources section (Chapter 16), I list a few places for you to get started.

How Can a Carnivore Diet Be So Helpful? What the Hell's Going On?

Because there's so little science, and the recent carnivore "movement" is so new, there's not much more than speculation at this point. If the diet is helpful, what is the reason? There are two main schools of thought.

1. A carnivore diet *eliminates bad stuff*. In particular, inflammatory foods (especially foods that people have not generally regarded as causing inflammation, i.e., certain plants, or plants in general).

2. A carnivore diet *adds good stuff*. Specifically, a shock-and-awe level of nutrient density that your body hasn't experienced since it was breastfeeding.

As Dr. Shawn Baker, the godfather of carnivore eating says, "Sometimes subtraction is better than addition."

An "elimination diet" is a method for identifying problematic foods, in which you "eliminate" almost everything and then add back one item at a time and see when the problem resumes. At its core, the carnivore diet is really just an easy elimination diet if you think about it. When eating a carnivore diet, one can quickly see what is harming versus helping. Meat is not a highly allergenic food, so by cutting out everything but meat, one can slowly add items back in and get a true sense of what foods are irritating.

I like long-term carnivore, Amber O'Hearn's (of Ketotic.org) description of a carnivore diet as a "minimum viable product." One can start with that. Then, what happens if that person starts adding a bowl of spinach each day (or kale, or tomatoes). Does it make the person feel better? Does it make the person feel worse?

And with meat being so delicious, it's the easiest elimination diet I've ever seen.

Humans, Meat, and Evolution

Experts say we evolved on a diet heavy in meat and fat. We ate meat and lots of it. And not just meat, but hearts, liver, spleens. Freakin' bone marrow sucked right out of the bone.

Does that mean we should eat strictly carnivore though? I don't know. What about our ancestors eating a handful of berries once in a while, some tubers, or some honey? After all, they weren't just hunters, they were hunters *and gatherers*, right?

Certainly. Primordial humans ate pretty much anything they could get their hands on. Their survival depended on adaptability, both over seasons as well as generations. In time, different peoples populated different parts of the world, with vastly different environments. Flint-spear-toting mammoth hunters of the Eurasian steppes clearly had a different diet than Polynesian islanders. Even today, some populations have a gene that lets them digest milk, whereas those without the gene are lactose-intolerant. Who's to say what's "best"?

To answer that question, consider what all humans and habitats have *in common*: They all have edible animals. Notably, they do not all have edible plants.

Look at it this way. Edible, non-poisonous greens and sweet, starchy foods during human prehistory were available perhaps only occasionally or seasonally, such that we evolved a *craving instinct*, to eat as much of them as we can find, in order to store them, primarily as fat reserves, for periods of low food availability. That same metabolic hoarding mechanism and craving instinct is still genetically hardwired into us, but now it's basically a deadly adaptation in a world of abundant, cheap, mechanized food production. Starches are not self-limiting! We stop ourselves from eating another delicious cookie only because we know we should stop (or if you're like some people, you don't stop until you run out of cookies). Food that requires discipline to *not eat* is not what we're supposed to be eating every day.

Meat, on the other hand... think about it... what happens when you've had your fill of meat? You simply stop. It's the self-limiting food. Unlike that second serving of pie or mashed potatoes that goes straight to your waistline, metabolically speaking, it does not require discipline to resist a second steak. Weird, right? For whatever reason from our biological past, we do not seem to be programmed to eat ourselves to death with meat. When we're done, we're done.

Also important to consider is the differences in plants we're eating today from those in ancient times. Our fruits and vegetables today have been hybridized and bred into unrecognizable versions of their ancestors, usually bigger and sweeter. That apple or orange you see today did not exist in the time when our genes were laid down on the African savannah.

According to some, we can get every nutrient we need, in the best possible format, from animal products. Meat is actually extremely nutritious. Dr. Georgia Ede, from DiagnosisDiet.com, notes:

"Meat is the only nutritionally complete food. Animal foods (particularly when organ meats are included) contain all of the protein, fat, vitamins and minerals that humans need to function. They contain absolutely everything we need in just the right proportions. That makes sense, because for most of human history, these would have been the only foods available just about everywhere on the planet in all seasons."

Another common sentiment in the carnivore community is that "*meat heals.*" My experience supports this, as do the experiences and testimonials of many others. Meat, especially *beef*, has super nutrition, without any of carbohydrates' negative consequences. For instance, many sources of seemingly innocent carbohydrates can be inflammatory, which a lot of people (and even most doctors) don't realize.

Plus, even though plants possess some nutrition, it's not always accessible or "bio-available." Eliminating plants from my diet, and replacing calories with nutrient-rich animals products like beef did wonders for my body in fortifying it and reducing inflammation. Perhaps it's all placebo effect, but I felt extra nourished the entire time, and subsequent times that I'm on a carnivore diet. And the great, lean, "nourished" feeling goes away just as soon as I start introducing other foods into my diet. Placebo or not, you don't have to try something very many times, and see the same result each time, to start recognizing that something is working for you. It seems to be in my case, so far, at least.

But Don't Just Take My Word for It

These are the kind of things I continue to ponder as I navigate my carnivore diet. You have to experiment with food on your own. Become the world's leading authority on what makes you feel great. Experiment. Keep a food journal. Take notes. Not only notes about what you eat, but how other things are going, such as strength/workouts, bowel movements, sleep, energy levels, and mood. (I deliberately do not ever step onto a scale or track my weight; the "mirror measurement" is sufficient and daily water fluctuation can make you crazier than a Bitcoin day trader.)

Some people will only find their best health, like Amber O'Hearn, mentioned above, by eating a zero carb carnivore diet. Others will find that after eating a carnivore diet for a period of time, they can add certain plants back in their diets without negative consequences, or without too much discomfort, or weight gain. At that point, you can decide if you want plants added for convenience or pleasure, and in what quantity and frequency.

Some carnivore dieters discover that they have previously unknown allergies to plants – perhaps even to the very phytonutrients that are supposed to be beneficial. For them, cutting out the allergens and irritants completely could be why they felt even better going carnivore instead of eating just low-carb or keto.

Another example, Charlene Andersen, who shared her story on MeatHeals.com, has been eating ribeyes and drinking spring water, exclusively, for *twenty* years. Seriously. She tried every diet you can think of while she was sick with various illnesses. As she cut carbs and increased fats, she improved, but she wasn't completely healed. But according to Charlene, when she went all-beef, every single one of her symptoms vanished. She looks fantastic, too, and she's in her mid-40s!

Some people might choose to eat a meat-only diet for some stretches of time, and at other times, to have some plants (maybe during the holidays or on vacations or simply just for the heck of it). These people will have to consider whether any deviation from a carnivore diet induces carbohydrate cravings or not. That's a common problem.

And others find they simply desire the extra restrictive diet, because they think it's the simplest, tastiest, most frugal, and most satisfying: beef and water.

I find it interesting that many people who were previously having success on a low-carb/keto diet had even more success after starting the carnivore diet. They felt there was room for improvement from the low-carb keto diet. They report that the low-carb diet was great for a while and helped them heal many ailments, but then they hit a plateau and it was no longer as effective. For example, after initially losing weight, some people started to slowly gain some weight back after a while of eating low-carb. Others felt the ailments were improved, but not completely healed. They longed for a better solution.

The person going from low-carb keto to "zero carb" carnivore allows a person to eat more protein and still stay in ketosis versus the typical ketogenic diet which makes room for some carbohydrates instead of the extra protein. The possible implications/benefits as to why many people could feel better on a carnivore diet versus a standard ketogenic diet (which has plants) could be that the higher protein makes them feel well, or is healing things. Or, it could be the elimination of even those small amounts of carbohydrates makes them feel better. Or, is it the plants that were the problem? Some experts think it's the plants (not the carbs, but rather, the wide range of phytonutrients) that are the problems, even in small amounts.

Bottom line: Eating a carnivore diet seems to be helping a lot of people both in the short term and long term.

CHAPTER 2: A SKEPTIC'S TALE: HOW I CAME TO TRY THE CARNIVORE DIET

Ever since moms have existed, we've been told to "eat your vegetables." It's so deeply ingrained in our belief systems that it sounds crazy to even question it, right? Like the sun rising every morning, or objects falling when you drop them.

Well, I'm no longer convinced "eat your vegetables" is good advice for everyone. When I was eating meat and vegetables – even really "healthy" vegetables (spinach, kale, etc.) – I still had my range of generic health issues. Everyone does, right? That's just part of life, right?

Maybe not. When I look back on my life, the times I ate more protein and fat, and fewer plants, for a long period of time, I felt better. In my early 20s, as a competitive bodybuilder eating a high protein diet low in plants, I felt great. I was also working out a lot. And I was young. I'm sure those helped. But still... what if?

As I mentioned previously, later on came the decade of my life where I ate a strict vegan diet. I started off feeling great. I believe this was because I was coming off a standard diet, and going vegan eliminated many crap foods. But after that initial honeymoon period, I started to not feel as well again. I was having too many headaches, we had fertility problems, there was that damn rash on my finger that would not go away no matter what I did, I had frequent nausea after eating, and I was getting painful cystic acne.

Yet I was blind to the idea that my personal health struggles could've been linked to my diet, because, after all, I thought the vegan diet was the best. But after a while, my body became depleted despite my taking great care to supplement properly, to the tune of hundreds of dollars a month. In hindsight, I was too vested in the vegan philosophy and lifestyle to admit it to myself. I thought it was anything other than my diet. Even worse, I had my husband, daughter, and mom on the vegan diet. I was terribly wrong. My family suffered.

Of course, I know more now about nutrition, scientific studies, and the risk of relying on observational studies. If I knew back then what I know now, then I would never have gone vegan. It was a big mistake and I paid the price.

After ending my vegan diet, I embraced a variety of omnivore styles, from Weston A. Price's *Real Food*, to Paleo, to Bulletproof. And sometimes I felt great. I had improvements in various health areas after ending the vegan diet, because I was finally getting the animal-based nutrients that my diet was lacking. With a diet rich in animal products plus some vegetables, I had more good days than bad. My acne dramatically improved, and I only had a few pimples once in a while. My headaches improved, though they didn't completely go away. My energy was decent, and on days that it was low, I blamed it on lack of exercise and the hardships of motherhood.

So, overall, I was doing quite well. I had heard of low-carb and keto diets and I wanted to experiment with one, but every time I did, it never lasted more than a few days. I think that having even just a few carbohydrates, or having to choose a small amount of carbs from the overwhelming range of choices, prevented my long-term success.

At that time, I had no idea there was an alternative. I didn't know people were actually cutting out ALL carbs and eating a carnivore diet. That would have sounded totally bonkers to me... humans aren't lions, right? But indeed there were people doing it. And they were starting to see some interesting results. I just hadn't heard about it yet.

My First Exposure to the Carnivore Diet

So, what prompted my "craziness" of not eating plants?

Enter: Shawn Baker, MD:

I learned about Dr. Shawn Baker when my friend, Ben, retweeted something from him about eating only meat. I chuckled at his *absurd* diet of eating as a carnivore. Who the fuck only eats meat? What a loon.

Hm. What's that? He's a doctor?...

That's right, Dr. Shawn is an MD promoting the awesomeness of eating a carnivore diet. I couldn't help but do a double take. He's an orthopedic surgeon no less. Well, that piqued my interest, seeing as most doctors are still touting the outdated idea of watching cholesterol consumption.

And, I'm a diet-curious gal.

I saw that he is a big dude! He is super muscular and in great shape for being 51 years old (he's in great shape for any age actually!). I found myself more entertained than anything. I started following him on Twitter, where his tweets at first seemed pretty drastic. I saw once that he was eating 8 plain hamburger patties for a meal. I thought, "Huh, that's... um, bizarre, funny, interesting, and possibly ridiculous."

Over the months, I saw his meaty meals posted on twitter, and saw him retweeting other people trying the carnivorous way.

Then, as I had done so many times before over the years, down the diet rabbit hole I went. From those initial intriguing links and blog posts, I read story after story from self-proclaimed "carnivores" and their fascinating experiences. Turns out there was an active Facebook group with over 11,000 followers (as of this writing). Some having done it for decades! Woah. *Decades?* Yes. Only meat for decades? Yes.

But I still wasn't really interested in doing it myself. Maybe in the deep recesses of my mind I ran a "what if" scenario, but I shut it down. We need our plants. Duh.

Then, Dr. Shawn Baker appeared on Joe Rogan's podcast. I really like Joe Rogan's podcast, and if someone makes it on there, well, Joe will at least make it very entertaining. I eagerly listened since I knew who Dr. Shawn Baker was and what he was about. I knew Joe Rogan would ask good, direct questions and I'd get the full story.

I found myself completely engrossed for the entire two-hour interview. I was suddenly going beyond the "what if" in the back of my mind to wondering what my husband would say if I started a carnivore diet today.

Dr. Shawn Baker addressed issues like pooping when there's no fiber in the diet, vitamin C and scurvy when the carnivore diet isn't high in vitamin C, strength gains, recovery in the gym, and much more.

I was becoming more interested, and I started thinking ahead to the dialogue I'd have with my husband. I'd lead with "strength gains in the gym and less inflammation." I'd hook him with that.

Next, I read more online about those common questions. Heck, I hadn't even thought of those myself back when I briefly wondered whether I would eat a carnivore diet.

I dug deeper and listened to interviews with scientists and researchers talking about how we don't actually need plants, and that we can get micro-nutrients from animals, along with the essential fatty acids and essential amino acids. I read that carbohydrates aren't essential. My mind was exploding. I couldn't devour these podcasts and interviews fast enough.

The experts talking about these topics said we need more research, and I completely agree. But that didn't change something important. Notably that there was currently NOT good science for the constant recommendation to eat more fruits and vegetables. Wow. At this point, I just switched to imagining how easy my life would be if I wasn't preparing any plants to eat every day.

Over time, I watched Dr. Shawn Baker with increasing fascination. I read about others and saw more impressive before-and-after photos of pre- and post-carnivore diet. There were people with full acne going to crystal-clear skin. There were people losing drastic weight. People were claiming increased energy, mood, sex drive, and overall happiness. All anecdotal, but impressive nonetheless.

Then, yet again, I put on my inch-thick skeptic glasses. I sensed disturbing familiarity, similar to the dietary cult-like worship I'd had when I was vegan, and that scared me. My mad scientist enthusiasm for weird and extreme diets (and sharing successes) is permanently tempered by my bad experience following the vegan herd years ago. I really tried to see and experience the carnivore diet in a different light, with smart curiosity, open eyes, no preconceived expectations, but also with...

... a healthy dose of skepticism.

So I set out to try and poke holes in the carnivore diet. I reminded myself that when someone drastically changes their diet and cuts out crap, it's very common to see great initial improvements, whether the new diet is vegan, keto, low-carb, whole-foods, real-food, vegetarian, or even carnivore. They also shout it from the rooftops, thinking they've finally found "the" answer.

So, yes, many people came from a crap diet and reported awesome health improvements after going carnivore. But here's where things started sounding different. It wasn't just SAD (standard American diet) people having improvements on a carnivore diet; there were people trying a carnivore diet coming from other "healthy" diets like keto, low-carb, real-food, and even they had surges in health coming from a starting point of already being pretty healthy. That was something new!

In my strong attempt to not be biased, I considered whether those mysterious, long-term carnivore dieters are simply steeped in their own meat-filled dogma, drinking their own beef broth-flavored Kool-Aid. Are they possibly ignoring problems that might actually be there, or chalking them up to something else? I was guilty of that as a long-term vegan. I found ways to explain away the facts that didn't fit my worldview. Are these crazy carnivores doing the same thing?

Despite my skepticism, I kept coming back to the same thought:

It can't hurt to try a carnivore diet for just a little while.

In line with the past 20 years of my life, where I loved experimenting with different ingredients and diets, always eager to see what improvements could be had, I wanted to give carnivore a try. Now I was really curious. I started creating my carnivore diet shopping list.

The Day I Pulled the Trigger

When I told my husband I was going to eat a carnivore diet, he too was understandably skeptical. But we've been married a long time and he's witnessed my crazy experiments and diverse diets. I don't think anything would surprise him at this point. He also knew I'd been researching the subject, so it wasn't a total shock to him. I'd been peppering our conversations with testimonials and anecdotes I was reading, plus facts and figures. He knew something was up before I said anything officially.

Him: But, really... carnivore?

Me: Yes.

Him: No plants?

Me: That's right.

I started with a simple 30-day goal. I saw no downside to eating no plants for a month, even if doing so for a week might seem radical to normal people. This was, after all, an experiment. *For science!* I wanted to see if I'd feel any different by eliminating plants from my diet, and I figured I needed to give it at least a month to feel anything change.

I was excited about eating a carnivore diet because I knew about the strong nutrition in meat and I wondered what benefits I might get by having so much. Meat contains a shit ton of micronutrients. Maybe we can thrive *without any plants. What if???*

I did question, for a while, whether eliminating plants would harm me. Were there any nutrients in plants I needed that I couldn't get from animals?

Turns out... no. However, one must consider the context. If someone is eating plants that include many in the form of refined carbohydrates, which have less nutrition than fruits and vegetables, then they would likely benefit from swapping those refined carbs for fresh produce. But, if I'm on a carnivore diet, the fruits and vegetables are not likely to contribute any new benefit, according to those that say meat has all the nutrients the human body needs.

However, if a person is ill or challenged with a particular disease, while a zero-carb carnivore diet might bring great health, I am not equipped to say that some plants, acting as medicines, would or would not help. Plants can have powerful medicinal benefits.

To be very clear: More quality studies need to be done on this way of eating. A carnivore diet breaks so starkly from the current conventional dietary rules that we actually know very little about them.

So again, we've all heard for ages about the need for vegetables? But, what if the conventional preachers were wrong? What if you only need phytonutrients in vegetables to counteract the deleterious effects of grains, for instance? Given the state of contradictory nutritional science, it's not too hard to find a study supporting anything you like. I don't have much confidence in the data we have for the truth of any diet. Until more, and better, studies are done, I'm happy to experiment on myself, and go down another dietary rabbit hole, always asking, "What if?"

Even as I write this, I'm still a skeptic though.

I still don't know whether it's best to only eat meat (protein and fat) and drink water versus including some animal by-products (high-fat dairy), or allow some "flex-meals"/"cheat days," or just the occasional handful of primeval berries. I just don't know. What I do know is that there are people eating a carnivore diet and they didn't drop dead from it. On the contrary, they seem to be flourishing. Or rather, that appears to be the case, as best we can tell from self-reported success stories (maybe there are failures who don't bother to share their stories... aka "survivorship bias"). It really does come down to the individual and their circumstances, their health, etc.

CHAPTER 3: MY RESULTS

I wasn't particularly sick or in ill health when I started. Before eating a carnivore diet, I was mindful of what I ate, but I wasn't overly restrictive except to say that I avoided all soy, overly processed vegetable oils (I did consume coconut oil and olive oil), and I did not eat anything that I consider to be "total crap," such as overly processed foods, fried foods, cereals, things with food colorings or synthetic chemicals, stabilizers, etc. I basically ate what people refer to as "whole" and "real" foods.

I felt mostly healthy, but I was a bit obsessed with food. I didn't want to stop at just one cookie so I avoided them entirely or I would be addicted. I had cravings from time to time which I induced willpower to get through (not fun). I occasionally had pimples, sometimes around my menstrual cycle. I experienced migraine headaches at times. I had occasional pain in my hip or I'd tweak something in my back on occasion, and it'd take longer than it seemed it should take to heal. My energy levels were moderate, but I had the usual stress of motherhood and lack of exercise contributing to that.

But I felt pretty good most days, and given the sorry state of modern society's nutrition and health, any doctor would say I was in great health compared to the average person. But when I ate a carnivore, diet I felt noticeably better in many ways.

Here is what I experienced:

I Was Not Hungry All Day

This was one of my favorite benefits. I used to think about food constantly, partly from a love and passion for food and partly from obsession. But after going carnivore, after finishing a 16-ounce ribeye steak for breakfast (yes, that's right), I felt great all day and didn't snack or even think about food until dinner time. I didn't obsessively think about food because everything was simplified (no planning required) and I could go hours between meals. I was completely satisfied. The cravings were gone.

It Was Super Easy

I really want to make this point because this was life-changing for me. Prior to eating a carnivore diet, my life included a lot of time in the kitchen. Lots of chopping, washing produce, making multiple meals a day.

That's all different on a carnivore diet. I spend so much less time with meal prep now that it's liberating. It's like a genie from a bottle just gave me an extra 1-2 hours a day to spend however I want.

Additionally, I don't have so many choices for food. Call it what you like – the Paradox of Choice, Paralysis by Analysis, Decision-Making Fatigue – it doesn't matter, it's a very real thing. When you strategically eliminate choices, you free up brain cycles for other stuff in your busy day. (Einstein famously wore the same colored clothes every day so that he could solve the universe instead of figuring out what to wear.) By not having to think through many options, everything is simplified. I'm fascinated that restricting my food choices would actually make me feel more free. Me and Einstein, life-hackin' bros.

I Didn't Crave Sugar or Carbs

I believe this is the main reason why so many people trying a carnivore diet are able to keep at it. For some people, having any carbs, even leafy greens, can induce sugar cravings. I can follow a carnivore diet without any effort because I don't think about carbohydrates. Bread and toast, two of my favorite things – these literally don't even cross my mind. If they come up randomly, I just have no desire for them, so long as I've had steak or eggs in the past few hours. It's not willpower. I usually eat two meals a day, with zero interest in snacks or food outside those meals. That is liberating!

That's not to say that carbs don't sound good when I'm hungry. When hungry, most anything sounds good. However, in those moments, if I think about my preference for a carnivore diet food versus anything with carbohydrates, I always want the animal food. In fact, when it comes to my birthday, I want nothing more than a big-ass ribeye steak with a candle in it.

I Finally Got to Experience the Benefits of Shifting Into Ketosis

I had read time and again about people eating a keto or low carb diet. The trouble was that I could never last on it. I was eager to experience energy derived ketogenically to see if my brain power increased and my energy went up. After hearing so many hardcore athletes rave about the nearly magical benefits, I wanted to experience some of that for myself.

But whenever I had tried doing that on a low-carb diet, I couldn't manage to stay on it long enough to experience the effects. I'm a woman with a lot of willpower. I can be very determined. However, even I struggled eating low-carb after doing it for a few days. I think this is the result of three things:

- It meant having "any" carbs, and that was still too many carbs for me.
- There was too much variety in the meals. It wasn't simple enough. Too many choices for my mind made me want more.
- It is possible that having any plants, on a regular basis, was harming my body, or at least causing me to crave more food.

It Was the Easiest Thing I've Ever Done to Stay in Great Shape

On a carnivore diet, I'm in the shape I had in my 20s. When I ate what I thought was a "clean" diet during the past decade of my life, sure, I stayed in good shape. But, I had to put a lot more effort into it. My muscles have taken on more definition and they're shapelier. That's without working out consistently. And, when I was able to work out consistently, gains came faster and lasted longer.

(Note: This is possibly due to the high levels of creatine in beef. If you seek gains in the gym, you'll want to make sure you're getting 5 grams of creatine a day. You can do this without supplementing if you consume 2 pounds of beef, three pounds of chicken, or 1.5 pounds of herring.)

I was stronger, too. I could do more pull-ups, which I've found to be a good barometer for my overall strength. More often than not, I felt like getting off my ass and banging out push-ups, sometimes multiple times a day. My plank time increased from 2 minutes to 3 minutes almost overnight.

Beautiful Skin

Ahhhhh the joy of having clear skin. *I love you, carnivore diet, for helping my skin stay clear of pimples 99% of the time.*

Contributing to great skin: My diet is way less inflammatory, my hormones are better balanced, and I'm getting more nutrition. Minor skin wounds seemed to heal faster.

I think the carnivore diet could also be anti-aging, but I haven't been on it long enough to tell. My skin texture is improving though. Further, the long-term carnivores look great, and it's probably from not eating sugars, combined with the boosted nutrition in meat.

(Note: I address skin and migraines in more depth in the next chapter, *Carnivore Diet for Women*.)

Hip Pain Improved

I've had hip pain for years since sleeping on one side for so long while pregnant. It used to wake me up many times each night, which affected other areas of my life. My hip started to get better when I ceased being vegan, but on occasion it would flare up. Now it bothers me way less. There is no daily soreness. If it bothers me at all, it's only after taking a 2 or 3-hour walk. Now I sleep through the night.

I'm not claiming my carnivore diet means never having a little ache or pain. I occasionally wake up with a sore neck or tweak my foot while walking. However, the discomfort is shorter lived than when I had plants in my diet, which I assume is due to reduced inflammation.

Fewer Headaches

My migraine attacks are much less frequent. I think stress is a great contributor to migraine headaches, as well as weather changes, etc., and so I don't expect to be headache-free completely. But I do expect a drastic reduction if I'm eating such a simple and pure diet. There are many migraine food triggers, mostly from the plant kingdom. Eliminating those triggers just had to reduce my migraines, and it did!

Mental Well-Being

Mentally, I feel amazing. (Ask my husband, he sees it every day.) I feel strong, empowered, just a bit happier, and with a little more spring in my step. It's probably part real (the nutrition) and part placebo.

I mean, who wouldn't feel like a badass eating huge steaks and tearing meat straight off the bone? Call me a wild girl.

No Bloating

My guts feel great. With a carnivore diet, I can go from eating a huge steak to wearing a swimsuit five minutes later, because I still have a flat tummy. There's zero bloating... it's kind of amazing. I love the feeling I get after eating a satisfying carnivore meal and not feeling a bit bloated. Vanity maybe? Sure. I don't care.

Expected Benefit: Dental Health

Want to hear something that's not controversial about carbohydrates and there's lots of research on? Sugar is bad for teeth. This is something even the "eat your vegetables" grannies and I can agree on!

It's a hot topic for me... excellent dental health became a passion (ok, an obsession), when my teeth went to hell from eating a vegan diet for a decade.

I think it's very possible that, in time, the carnivore diet will be determined to be one of the best ways for building and maintaining healthy teeth. For me, that means including things like sardines (with bones), getting sunshine, fatty fish and pork fat (for vitamin D), and including some quality cheeses, eggs, and/or liver (for vitamin K2 and retinol).

In Conclusion...

For the short term, I've been eating a carnivore diet I've experienced great benefits. They're enough to keep me sticking with it. I don't know what will happen for me long term if I can keep it up, but based on other long-term carnivore dieters' experiences, I'm optimistic that I could have a lot to look forward to.

Sidebar: My Husband's 2-Week Experiment With the Carnivore Diet

My husband's story provides a good example for my disclaimer that "your mileage may vary." It also might suggest some pitfalls to avoid.

He went carnivore for two weeks. It was not long enough to claim any benefits with any confidence, but he described two "very promising" indicators.

1. Strength

As he relayed it to me, "You know that feeling in the gym, when you go to put a 45-lb plate on the bar, and it feels lighter the moment you pick it up? And you already know you're going to have a good benchpress? It was like that, probably after about a week. Every day."

2. Shoulder Pain Decreased

Like every gym vet over 40, my husband has had his share of shoulder injuries. One particularly bad one had him in physical therapy and no benchpress (or even pushups) for over a year, but it wasn't quite bad enough to warrant surgery, either. Nothing but time healed it. But eventually, he was able to do careful bench exercises with no pain. His shoulder is mostly better now, but he's extremely cautious, and finely attuned to any slight discomfort, and then he backs off. It's a limiter on potential gains, because he won't push beyond a certain level of pain, which is where the gains are to be found.

Well, after two weeks of eating nothing but beef, he told me one day "my shoulder feels great, like I never injured it." He was able to start attempting heavier weights than he had in years, without the slight tinge that told him to stop.

Those were the good results. Now the bad.

Cravings

In the two weeks, my husband never lost his cravings for carbs. He wanted "something else" (carbs) even after eating a huge steak and his stomach was literally "full." He said the entire two weeks felt like when he had done an intense low-calorie fast for some fast weight loss several months earlier. During his fast, he became "comfortable with hunger," but it was hunger nonetheless, abated somewhat by appetite suppression via decaf coffee throughout the day. He was still feeling this "hunger" feeling eating all the beef he could stomach. I never experienced anything remotely like this.

Why the Difference? Possible Reasons

1. Not Long Enough

It's very possible that his body simply didn't transition to a ketogenic metabolism as quickly as mine presumably did. Perhaps if he had given it a couple more weeks, the cravings would have gone away.

2. Not Enough Fat

I eat all the fat that comes on the steak, and I don't trim any off before I cook it. My husband is still grossed out by eating a big blob of greasy fat. He eats much more fat than he used to, but still leaves some fat on the plate. He gets plenty of butter (that too, was an adjustment, after years of brainwashing about the evils of fat), but it's very possible that he wasn't getting enough calories. He says that if he were to try carnivore again, he would try to eat more fat.

3. Not Strict Enough

Halfway into his carnivore experiment, one night my husband felt sick to his stomach. The thought of eating anything meat-related made him want to throw up. He ate some bread to settle his stomach, and the nausea instantly went away. I'm not sure about the cause of the nausea (could've been anything), but this load of carbs midway through might have reset his metabolism back to square one, delaying any transition to ketosis.

So let these serve as a potential warning. If you decide to try the carnivore diet, you might want to:

- Do it long enough to change your metabolism
- Eat LOTS of fat, and then some
- Don't cheat. I've outlined some approaches where people can "ease into" the carnivore diet, but be aware that these half-measures might make it harder to reach the goal.

As we travel abroad, my husband is currently on a high-meat diet, but not carnivore. He feels that when he's consuming large portions of beef, he may be experiencing many of the carnivore diet benefits, though it's hard to tell for sure, as our travels have made it difficult to do regular resistance training.

CHAPTER 4: CARNIVORE DIET FOR WOMEN (OR THE WOMAN IN YOUR LIFE)

I wrote the first edition of this book to share with both men and women what I had learned and experienced eating a carnivore diet. However, as a woman who has eaten this way for almost a year now, I've noticed benefits specific to women that I want to share. Furthermore, over the past few months, as the carnivore diet has started to get more awareness, I've come to learn that there are quite a few women enjoying experiences ⊠similar to mine.

Canaries in My Coal Mine

I have a few personal warning indicators for how my health is going. The canaries in my coal mine, if you will, are:

- Pimples
- Migraines
- PMS

When one or more of these is flaring up, I feel it's a sign that something is out of balance and it could be causing all kinds of additional problems that I can't see.

I feel like the converse is also true: When my skin is clear, I've had no headaches in weeks, and my periods are a breeze, I can pretty much assure you that everything else health-wise is going great, too.

Keep these three canaries in mind as I relay some of my experiences, below.

(Once upon a time, I would have added "low energy" to my canary list, but when you're a stay-at-home, world-traveling, indie-author, homeschooling mom, all bets are off. Laying down to bed at night with that "just run over by a truck" feeling is par for the course, no matter what you eat. That said, I definitely have more energy in general when I m eating zero/low-carb.)

Is a Fit and Flat Tummy Too Much to Ask?

I admit it — I like having a flat tummy. Always have, always will. However, my passion for a flat tummy is dashed when I eat plants. Back when I was 20 and a competitive bodybuilder, I used to complain to my coach about my stomach sticking out after eating. He used to say, "⊠Girl, it s just food. ⊡" I had another friend tell me that, because of my narrow waist, my stomach had to stick out after eating because the food didn't have anywhere to go. This pacified me briefly, but I still wasn't very comfortable and I never liked it.

Fifteen years later, there I was, still complaining about it to my husband. He repeated the same thing my former coach and friend did, ⊠"Honey, you just ate. It's food."⊠ Now, in my early 40s, I'm eating a carnivore diet, and something very interesting has happened…

From Steak to Swimsuit

It wasn't long before I realized one of my favorite things about a carnivore diet: I can eat a huge freakin' steak and, when I'm done eating, I'm not bloated. WHAT??? Yes. Finally!

I'll never forget the day I realized that I wasn't bloated after eating over a pound of delicious ribeye. The weather was hot and my daughter wanted to go to the pool. Ordinarily, I'd want to wait a couple of hours after eating before strutting about in a swimsuit by the pool, but I realized I could happily don my bikini right then. I had just eaten a pound of steak! Nothing remained on my plate but the bone. And you'd never know that I d just enjoyed all of those delicious calories by looking at my flat tummy.

I felt energized and ready to go do anything. A big, fatty, satisfying steak seems like a lot of food, and I suppose it is. A pound of meat is not what you normally see on a woman' s plate, or even a hungry man' s. But here I was, eating a huge freakin' slab of meat twice a day and I was amazed that I never got bloated. Now, I can' t help but question all the times I tried telling myself that being bloated after eating was natural and OK. Well, it wasn't OK for me.

This Carnivore Diet Kept Coming Up Roses for Me

I was really excited about my consistently flat tummy on a carnivore diet. But it turns out that eating only meat was great for a host of reasons beyond just a flat tummy. I felt energized, focused, and I wanted to work out and move my body more. Then, I learned how easy the diet was to maintain, and how much more time I had as a result. That' s always good for us mamas.

Carnivore Skin Health vs. Being a Wrinkly Vegan

When the lightbulb went on for me in my mid-30s and I questioned the validity of my decade of eating a vegan diet, I looked down at my knees one day. I was dismayed to see the skin on them was sagging. I was like, ⊠*WTF, old knees?!* There was no reason for my knee skin to be sagging. I was in my fucking 30s. I exercised all the time. I was supposedly eating the healthiest diet there was.

I immediately went to the bathroom and inspected my face. And my butt. In that moment, I realized that beyond a shadow of a doubt, my vegan diet had contributed to my aging faster than I should have. I was a non-smoker, I came from strong genes, I didn't eat crap processed foods. Yet here I was, aging faster than the Gilligan's Island folks when that meteor hit the island. Saggy knees, floppy hollow ass, and thinning skin on my face. Goddammit.

Animal Foods for Beauty

Guess what? When I changed my diet to include meat, eggs, and fish — almost immediately — I noticed a change. My rapid aging seemed to slow, but I had lost a lot of time. In my new (at the time) omnivore diet, I was automatically eating fewer carbs and including more nutritious skin-healthy foods. My natural olive-tone skin was revived from the ashen-gray tone it had taken on while eating vegan. My face filled out, and my ass stopped sagging like a 70-year-old's. I'd say that my vegan-intensified face wrinkles improved (maybe from proper hydration and my face filling out), but they didn't all go away, of course, because that damage was done. But on the whole, I was starting to look and feel much better.

The best I could hope for was that I was now on the right track. I hoped that my new diet with better foods would slow future aging. At this point, I wasn't even eating carnivore. I can' t say for sure how eating carnivore long-term will slow my aging even more, but when I started to read the information I'll convey below, it gave me even more cause for hope.

One thing was immediately certain: My skin cleared up from pimples when I went carnivore. I had experienced something similar when I went omnivore, but carnivore took it to new, unprecedented levels.

Sugar Steals Beauty

Sugar and carbohydrates are not good for your skin. They trigger inflammation, which can quickly result in acne, rashes, and other skin problems like accelerated aging. Those pesky sugar molecules attach themselves to protein fibers in our cells, and the damaging process (known as "glycation") results. Glycation limits the power of collagen to rebuild the skin s structure, increases the rate at which collagen breaks down, and robs your skin of its natural moisturizer, hyaluronic acid. I used to spend a lot a money on face products that contained hyaluronic acid. To think I could've saved all that money by just eliminating sugar. Many experts regard glycation as problematic for your skin as smoking and sun exposure. In fact, glycation makes the effects of smoking and sun damage even worse. Want accelerated wrinkly, saggy, dry skin? Eat carbs and sugars.

Carnivore Foods for Powerful, Effortless, Anti-Aging Beauty

The carnivore diet is a way of eating that eliminates accelerated-aging foods and amps up anti-aging foods.

Zinc and Carnosine

On a carnivore diet, I eat nutrient-rich foods like beef, fish, and chicken, which contain zinc and carnosine. Zinc is excellent for healing wounds and carnosine is shown to protect against advanced aging.

Omega-3 Fatty Acids for Fighting Skin Inflammation

If you eat fish (sardines are awesome!) then you re also enjoying an anti-inflammatory health boost with omega-3 fatty acids. The carnivore diet also reduces omega-6 fatty acids, which can cause inflammation.

Retinol for Acne and Wrinkles

Last but not least, there s retinol, which you get in egg yolks and liver. Now, I don t eat nearly as much liver as I should, but I do eat eggs. Retinol can do wonders for your skin. Heck, people are buying retinol in beauty products. Watch what happens to your skin when you consume it directly in food.

Bone Broth Is Bonafide Beauty Food

When you look at the nutrients that make up bone broth, you should expect delayed wrinkles, reduction in cellulite, stronger teeth, and glowing skin. Dr. Kellyann Petrucci uses bone broth to help her dangerously obese patients take off hundreds of pounds and to help Hollywood celebrities smooth their wrinkles and sculpt perfect bodies. And, according to Donna Gates, author of Body Ecology, bone broth can help decrease the appearance of cellulite and make your skin more supple and smooth-looking. Bone broth contains a number of nutrients, including collagen, that help build strong and beautiful skin.

Carnivore Diet as Skin Food

By eating a carnivore diet, you're eliminating sugar and carbohydrates, which we've just seen are extremely damaging to the skin. You' re also not eating inflammatory foods on a carnivore diet, and so you r skin will have less inflammation in the form of pimples, rashes, and other skin irritations. With bone broth, beef, eggs, and fish ⊠all common in a carnivore diet, plus the elimination of carbohydrates and sugars, you' re set to have the most amazing, glowing, clear and youthful skin of your life. I don t look like I m 22 (yet - haha), but I m certain the longer I eat this way, the better my skin will be.

PMS and Monthly Cycles on a Carnivore Diet

My experience with PMS has been all over the place for the past 20 years. Some cycles are a breeze and others are a total train wreck, with migraines, hormonal acne, water retention, and cramps. What I've found, however, is that on a carnivore diet, my cycle is the easiest. I've had months where I wasn't even expecting it and it came on so gently it surprised me. Where was the migraine? Where were the pimples? Where was the water retention? Over the course of almost a year eating carnivore, it took a few cycles to get to this point of PMS-greatness, as my hormones adjusted. I m not claiming it s all unicorns and glitter, but it s way easier than it used to be. This can be life-changing for so many women.

Over the year, each subsequent cycle seemed easier and easier. I remember last year, before I was on a carnivore diet, I even started logging my headaches because I was getting PMS headaches so regularly. It was becoming a pain, literally and figuratively. The weird thing is that it s not like my pre-carnivore diet was crap food. I was eating a healthy, whole-food diet with plenty of salads, Bulletproof Coffee, homemade organic sourdough bread, vegetables, meats, etc. I wasn't shutting myself in a closet eating Twinkies and Kit-Kats. Still, I had those fairly routine hormonal migraines. But then I went carnivore and, lo and behold, my migraines ceased in their regularity. They became infrequent, to the point that now I rarely get one. Everything about PMS improved for me.

That s where I am today. If the low rate of headaches and the health of my skin and PMS are any indication of my broader health, then that paints a good picture. My canaries are chirping happily!

I'm not saying that eating a carnivore diet will cure everything for everyone. I m not saying that I ll never get a pimple or a headache. But, damn, it' s close. I've never experienced anything like this in my adult years. And I've seen enough women eating a carnivore diet experiencing the same things to know it' s not just me.

Carnivore Pregnancy

I m not a doctor, but I ll share that I've read about women who've eaten a carnivore diet while pregnant. Of course, that' s something for you and your doctor to discuss, but the carnivore diet is new (well, ancient, but new to us) and I honestly wouldn't expect much support from your doctor if you tell him or her that you only eat meat while pregnant. There's not enough research for your doctor to provide much guidance without risking legal liability. Not to mention mere cultural bias… this is cray-cray territory to the less intrepid among us, and doctors are people, too. I personally don't think eating carnivore is crazy, but I also can't promise that it's safe. Either for you in the long-term, or for your baby in the short-term. It's a bit like venturing into the unknown.

Do your own research and listen to your own body. You can read about Kelly Hogan and how she has been on a carnivore diet for years, including pregnancy.

Does Going Zero-Carb (or Low-Carb) Negatively Impact a Woman' s Hormones?

It's anecdotal, but I've experienced nothing but great results eating a carnivore diet. It s been a little less than a year for me, but there are women out there who have eaten carnivore much longer than I have, and it s the only diet they've found that works for them.

While I think we can all benefit from consuming fewer carbs, I m not arrogant enough to say that everyone should eat zero carbs. Everyone is different and you'll have to experiment and see what works best for you. I have a friend who swears she needs carbohydrates for a healthy PMS cycle. To each her own; I found what works for me and it is, without a doubt, the carnivore diet as of now. I can't say for sure what I'll think as I age and experience hormonal changes through menopause and beyond, but I'm hopeful that a carnivore diet will continue to treat me well.

CHAPTER 5: FAQ: FREQUENTLY ASKED QUESTIONS ABOUT THE CARNIVORE DIET

What About Vitamin C, Magnesium, and Antioxidants? Can You Get These in a Carnivore Diet and Do You Need Them?

When I first heard about the carnivore diet, I kept thinking back to my fifth-grade history class when we learned about how sailors' teeth used to fall out and then they'd die, until Captain Cook made them eat lemons and, voila, that fixed it. Am I going to die of scurvy on a carnivore diet?

I feel the need to repeat that I'm not a nutritionist and this is not nutritional advice. But I will share some of the information I came across while considering a carnivore diet for myself. (There's a lot to say on this, and I recommend looking at the Resources section, Chapter 16, where you can find links to more information on what some scientists and researchers are saying.)

To begin, the history of how the government created the Recommended Daily Allowances (RDA) of various nutrients is highly suspect from a modern perspective. They created a blanket recommendation for the population, when in reality, vitamin and mineral requirements should be considered based on their diet and other factors (age, weight, activity level, etc.). We now know that, metabolically, carbohydrates cause the body to require different nutrients than diets that don't have carbohydrates. The implication is that, if you don't eat carbs, you don't need the same amounts of nutrients.

Amber O'Hearn explains more about vitamin C and the carnivore (ketogenic) diet.

"Given that a ketogenic metabolism uses different metabolic pathways and induces cascades of drastically different metabolic and physiological effects, it would be astonishing if any of the RDAs are entirely applicable as is."

I strongly suggest <u>reading more about her thoughts</u> on the matter to learn more about vitamin C and a ketogenic diet like a carnivore diet.

Currently, it seems that a lot of carnivore dieters don't typically take supplements, but that's entirely up to the individual and based on their circumstances. For example, there may be some caveats perhaps… stress levels of the individual, current health status, current ability to assimilate nutrients, current health goals, etc. It's also possible that someone on a carnivore diet won't take supplements for months or years and then later decide to.

In general, the consensus in the carnivore community is that a healthy person should be able to get everything they need from a carnivore diet if they're consuming adequate calories and getting plenty of them from beef. Some people recommend a small serving of offal, liver in particular, to get a vitamin boost. Some people like Dr. Shawn Baker, however, don't take any supplements and don't eat offal either. They also don't have scurvy or magnesium deficiencies.

Additionally, the vitamins and minerals in animal products are better absorbed than from plants. That's because, in plants, the fiber and anti-nutrients (phytates) make them less bioavailable.

I experienced this sad fact first-hand, when I was eating a vegan diet. Dr. Shawn Baker elaborates that plant-based diets drive up the nutrient requirements for people, and also make nutrients harder to assimilate, as they require more conversions and more work. To make matters worse, some people don't even have the ability to convert certain nutrients. Consider, for instance, the large part of the population who can't assimilate vitamin A from beta carotene in plants. Instead, they need it in the preformed retinol form from animal products. That was definitely my family and me.

Conversely, eating a meat-based diet lowers your requirements of certain nutrients and makes them more bioavailable at the same time.

What About Antioxidants? Don't We Need Those?

So how about those antioxidants? Again, Dr. Shawn Baker:

"Humans have a robust endogenous antioxidant system and it is upregulated when we reduce carbohydrate consumption."

And how about the phytochemicals we hear everyone discussing? For so many years I thought I was doing my body good by eating those phytonutrients (plant compounds). But check out this truth of phytochemicals: Polyphenols from plants are chemicals produced by plants to protect the plant, such as by making them poisonous to insects. In other words, some phytonutrients are literally insecticides. They may have medicinal relevance to humans, but to me, the argument that we need such compounds to be healthy, in this light, takes on an extra high burden of proof.

The words "polyphenol" or plant "nutrients" seem sexy. But, call them a plant's defense mechanism or nature's chemicals or plant toxins and they're more suspicious.

Phytochemicals work in various ways to protect the plant from being eaten. An animal's defense is running away or claws or teeth. A plant's defense is in these compounds we've long been told were helpful for us. They might not be. They actually could be harmful.

Dr. Georgia Ede writes:

"We are told that vegetables are powerful and virtuous... Yet vegetables have a dark side. They don't want to be eaten any more than animals do, and they use sophisticated chemical weapons to defend themselves…

"Because we believe that vegetables are good for us, we spend lots of time, energy, and money trying to prove how these bitter pesticides might be beneficial to human health. Because many of these same chemicals function as

"antioxidants" in the laboratory, scientists enjoy studying how they might be used to fight cancer and other diseases. ... wouldn't it make sense to also wonder whether these chemicals might be harmful to us?"

How Much Do I Need to Eat?

Well, how hungry are you? A great rule of thumb for the carnivore diet – since it's very hard to eat too much – is simply letting your appetite guide you. The simplicity of the food choices on a carnivore diet can help regulate one's hunger and appetite. Sometimes having so much variety encourages overeating.

That said, in the beginning, a common mistake among carnivore newbies is actually not eating enough. They're not used to eating so much meat and therefore they don't eat adequate amounts. Energy levels suffer a bit. As Dr. Shawn Baker is known for saying, "Eat meat like it's your job."

A transition tip: if you're not ready for a full carnivore diet yet, you could eat meat first at a meal, and try eating enough until satisfaction. After that, you could eat some plants to top off.

As a woman who is moderately active, I'm satisfied most days with about 1½ to 2 pounds of beef a day.

Dr. Shawn Baker says most people will find they are satisfied with that same amount (1½ to 3 pounds), but if you're an athlete or working out a lot, then you might do better eating up to 4 pounds of meat a day. Dr. Shawn Baker has even had days where he eats up to 6 pounds of ribeye a day. He's a big man, an athlete, and puts a lot of demands on his body. Anyone trying a carnivore diet needs to do their own experimenting to see what is most satisfying and gives them enough energy, calories, and nutrition. I found it helpful to read the various testimonials of other carnivores in finding my own way.

Can I Drink Coffee or Tea on a Carnivore Diet?

Coffee is a no-carb, zero-calorie plant extract. It should be considered a drug, not a food. Many carnivore dieters still drink coffee. I drink coffee, but ideally only on days when I'm writing or traveling. I also desire it more in cold months, so coffee intake is somewhat seasonal for me.

One great aid to reducing coffee consumption is drinking bone broth, especially during cold weather. Broth has no caffeine, but it's delicious, comforting, and very nutritious.

Do People Poop When Eating a Carnivore Diet?

Yes. Many carnivore dieters actually poop daily. Some people might skip a day here and there. For most carnivores, heck, maybe all… it's the best pooping experience ever.

The difference is the poop tends to be smaller and easier to excrete because it's not bulked up with fiber from plants. Meat is well absorbed by the small intestine, whose job it is to extract nutrition from food and put it in the bloodstream to use. The large intestine soaks up what's left (which isn't much on a carnivore diet), and prepares it for excretion.

Even better, flatulence is greatly reduced (basically non-existent!) when eating a carnivore diet. That's helping the environment, too, at least locally. :)

What Can I Eat at Restaurants?

If I know I'm going to a restaurant, I try to find the menu online beforehand. I might even call and ask questions, as detailed below, to arrange things before I arrive.

I pick out the meat dishes on the menu to consider. Then, I ask the server what they would charge for a meat-only dish.

For example, if a restaurant has a burger, I'll ask for a price of the patty only. If they come back with a price that is less than what I'd have paid for the whole thing (bun, condiments, sides), then yay! I'll order 2 or 3 of those patties.

However, if they don't offer a cheaper price for just the patty versus getting the bun etc, I'll ask if they can offer me a deal to get three patties by themselves. When I increase the number of patties and don't want any bread or sides, they are more willing to come down on the price per patty.

Sometimes a restaurant has a big steak, so I'll just order that and ignore the sides that come with it or tell them to leave the sides off.

For fast-food restaurants, I get beef patties only (pictured above, from In & Out) or patties with cheese only. There are some restaurants that have these options on a "secret" menu like In & Out (it's called the "Flying Dutchman"... and you can now consider yourself one of "those in the know."). Some carnivore dieters also like Wendy's because they sell all-beef patties only, and you can get them topped with bacon. While I don't make visits to fast food restaurants a regular habit, they have saved my butt in a pinch. I'd also visit them more when road tripping. After all, it's beef.

At Chipotle Mexican Grill, I get what I call a "carnivore bowl," which is just multiple servings of meat. I've done a mix of the chicken and steak, but I usually just prefer 3 servings of the steak.

Lastly, if I'm going to a restaurant, and I'm not sure I'll be able to eat enough food to get full (without breaking the bank), I'll eat some food before going so that I can eat a smaller portion of something at the restaurant. Conversely, I'll eat something at the restaurant, and if I'm still hungry I'll eat more once I'm home.

Do People Need Fiber?

I'm particularly fond of HighSteaks.com's discussion on the matter where it reads,

"I'm used to the disbelief and rage whenever I mention that fiber isn't essential, I get it, you grew up being accosted with the 'fact' that fiber is good for you and it does all these magical things. Frankly, they are nearly all completely wrong, and you've been led up the high-fiber garden path for too long, but nobody likes the idea that fiber might not be the mystical unicorn-grade asshole cleanser with god-like powers. The simple idea that we should be filling our digestive systems with something indigestible is utter madness."

We're told to eat fiber. Yet, interestingly, fiber can be irritating for many, many people. Why is fiber recommended in the first place? One argument is that it helps blunt blood sugar when eating carbohydrates. Well, if I don't eat carbohydrates then it would stand to reason that I don't need fiber. Eating fiber is an answer for a challenge that I don't have.

Fiber creates bulk, which can actually make it harder to poop. When your poop is smaller because it's not bulked up with fiber, it's usually easier to get out. There's less straining and that person is happy because they're not spending unnecessary time on the toilet.

According to Dr. Georgia Ede:

"At worst, fiber causes constipation, irritation and damage to the inner lining of the intestine, flatulence and pain."

And:

"We cannot digest the carbohydrates that make up soluble fiber ... Undigested carbohydrate fibers arriving in the colon attract huge numbers of bacteria for a free lunch. Is there anything wrong with that? ... bacteria don't exactly digest these carbohydrates, they ferment them, and in the process, they give off gases, like carbon dioxide, hydrogen, and methane ... they can also cause uncomfortable cramping and bloating, both common sense signs of poor digestion. Listen to your body: good digestion should not hurt. In contrast, animal protein and fat are comfortably and efficiently digested by humans with virtually no gases produced."

Some people question whether the microbiome would be negatively impacted from not eating fiber and plants, the things that feed it. To begin, we simply don't know enough about this area of science, and hopefully we will learn more, as it's a hot topic.

Amber O'Hearn thought-provokingly suggests, *"Evolutionarily, it would be implausible that any strain that couldn't stay alive without constantly feeding it would've been important to our bodies."*

Is Grass-Fed Meat Important?

For the animals, sure. I don't expect they enjoy the crowded feedlots where they are finished with grain before slaughter. Personally, I don't like the thought of them crowded in a lot eating the corn. I'd rather they get harvested in the field while eating grass, with harp music playing, but that's not realistic either.

However, paying a premium for grass-fed meat is not a smart financial choice for many. I wouldn't let the desire for grass-fed meat dictate whether I could eat a carnivore diet.

According to Dr. Shawn Baker, the vegan propaganda featuring animals (specifically cows) suffering is not the norm on farms. Most cows eat in pastures and most ranchers take care of their animals. For those instances where abuse has occurred, it's awful and should be stopped immediately. But, don't think that the beef you eat, which isn't labeled as grass-fed, meant the cow didn't eat grass. It did, and for much of its life. It's just often "finished" on corn (i.e., fattened up before slaughter). We should all strive to ensure animals aren't suffering, but most farmed animals are not.

Also, don't assume your source of beef suffered. The life cycle of domesticated animals is far less violent than the life of an animal in the wild. Going vegan is not the answer to what vegans would tell you about animals suffering. Interestingly, the monocropping that feeds vegans is destroying entire ecosystems and kills plenty of animals and insects on a regular basis. As Amber O'Hearn stated, "Life feeds on life. In order for me to live, other things have to die."

Can Kids Eat a Carnivore Diet?

As always, check with your doctor. That saying applies to you, and even more so for your kids. For one, their bodies are still developing, and their needs are different than adults'. But also, kids might not be as attuned as you are to what "feels" right or wrong. You've had a lot more years of experience, and you're not still growing. They also might not know to alert you if something changes.

It's been reported that children on medical ketogenic diets are more likely to get kidney stones. The carnivore diet is not the same as the keto diet, so it's unclear if this risk applies. Discuss this with your child's doctor. And if a doctor prescribes a therapeutic ketogenic diet for your kid, you could inquire as to whether that ketogenic diet could or should be meat-based and plant-free.

Some carnivore diet "experts" (including medical doctors) say yes, the carnivore diet is safe and healthy for children. However, it might be unrealistic to expect kids to adhere to it at all times. In some carnivore families, the kids eat mostly carnivore inside the home, and when outside the home they include plants for convenience and social norms (i.e., parties, etc.).

I'm not personally endorsing this, or any other, position on kids and the carnivore diet. I don't think we know enough yet. And even if we knew a lot more that's a discussion for you, your child (if he or she is old enough), and your doctor.

But I will report that there are testimonials of families who've tried it. See the Resources section (Chapter 16) for details.

One note of caution: All diets (and lifestyles) outside the mainstream have a long history of spooking authorities, who are understandably conservative when it comes to dealing with unknowns and children's welfare. It's their job and I don't hold it against them, because there are some dangerous people out there. But this means the authorities tend to be suspicious of anything that isn't officially endorsed by the usual Three Letter Acronym authorities or the relevant government agencies. If authorities receive a report or complaint about a child on a carnivore diet, they may be legally required to investigate, and they may feel compelled to intervene. Proceed at your own risk. Post on social media at very high risk.

One thing I do feel comfortable recommending is to encourage your kids to eat their meat. And probably more of it. And less grain-based carbohydrate, if they currently eat a lot. These suggestions are not controversial enough to cause concern for anybody.

CHAPTER 6: TIPS FOR TRANSITIONING TO THE CARNIVORE DIET

Transitioning to a carnivore diet was not difficult for me. In fact, it was one of the easiest things I've ever attempted. It felt more like I was shifting into something that felt more natural. I was also excited to try it, so that excitement fueled my motivation. I loved the food, I felt satisfied, I was feeling great despite a bit of "keto-flu" (see below). In this chapter, I'll share some tips for what made it an easy transition for me.

I'd say that I hear both sides when it comes to the ease or difficulty of transitioning to a carnivore diet. Many say it was easy mostly because they love beef, cheese, and bacon so much. Others have a tough time the first 3 to 10 days.

My first thought is it really depends on the motivation and excitement for trying it. My mom doesn't love the taste of most meats and it was harder for her. My husband does love meat and so it was easier for him.

For me, I loved the food and I surrounded myself with an online community of others trying it, which furthered my excitement. However, the good sleep I was getting, the clear skin I was immediately noticing, and the ease of the diet were motivators, too.

Essentially, I think this depends on where you are coming from with respect to diet, whether you're excited about the change, and whether you're implementing some transition tips. If you're coming from a diet high in carbohydrates, especially refined ones, then it could be a tougher transition for you. I'd expect to experience more "keto-flu" symptoms as your body adapts to eliminating carbohydrates, and replacing them with a lot more fat and protein.

If you're coming from a cleaner diet, or even a low-carb diet, already, then the likelihood of experiencing keto-flu is lower.

What Is the Keto-Flu? (aka Carb-Flu)

This is where someone might experience flu-like symptoms: tired, headache, aches, cranky, etc. The body goes through changes as it adapts to fat-burning and it isn't always fun. You can expect fluctuations in appetite, energy, and focus levels during that first week (or two, or three!). Things should eventually return to normal.

My own experience with keto-flu, coming from a Real-Food "clean" diet, was pretty minimal. I was more tired the first 3 days. I had a headache too, but I can't say for sure if this was due to the change in eating versus a sinus headache caused by something else.

There are things that can help reduce the keto-flu symptoms or make them less noticeable. Here are some options:

Ease Into It Slowly

One way to reduce the severity of the keto-flu symptoms, as well as just the mental adjustment, is simply ease into it gradually. Instead of going cold-turkey, start by making all breakfasts carnivore. After a week, make all breakfasts and lunches carnivore. Wait another week and make all breakfasts, lunches, and dinners carnivore.

This is just a sample; obviously, there are other schedules and ways to ease into it slowly. Feel free to get creative. Another way might be to start cutting out refined carbs from all meals first. Then, swapping grains with fruit and vegetables. Then, moving to all meat, etc.

Personally, I'm a cold-turkey kind of gal. Once I hear about something, I seek the benefits and experience immediately. It becomes an intense upfront learning curve, but I like that. Going cold-turkey was great for me, but I made sure to have enough meat and cheese in the house at all times.

Start on a Weekend or Vacation

You might prefer to start a carnivore diet during a time when you don't have to work or don't have intense obligations for other things. This could mean on the weekend, or better yet, on a long weekend away from work. This way, if there are keto-flu symptoms, they're easier to tolerate.

On the other hand, some people might prefer the distractions of work.

Allow More Time for Sleep

Although I found myself immediately needing less sleep, even from the first night, it's wise to at least allow for the extra rest. A nap might be in order during the first few days of transition.

Have the Right Expectations

If this is a dramatic change, then it could be both dramatically great and bad at the same time through the transition period. The greatness of losing weight, combined with the crappiness of being tired or having headaches.

Expectations don't stop with the carnivore dieter though. If you're embarking on the carnivore diet and you live with family or friends, then it's a good idea to help them have proper expectations, too.

My favorite way of approaching this is to tell others I'm trying something new to feel better and to please give me support. Sometimes simply asking for support is all a person needs to disarm the deniers. Understanding where these people are coming from is helpful too. If people don't support the diet, it's usually fear-based (which is really just ignorance in most cases) or jealousy. If it's based on ignorance, you could present helpful information as to why the carnivore diet might be a great choice. If it's based on jealousy, well, maybe enlisting the person to do it together is a tactic.

Either way, I find that simply asking for support straight up is a great way for people to be on the carnivore dieter's side.

Other considerations: People, understandably, thought I was crazy when I said I was eating a carnivore diet, and I'm even known for doing unconventional things. I wholeheartedly admit, I thought it was ridiculous the first time I heard it, too. I've spent the past 20 years of my adult life worshipping vegetables, whether I was omnivore or vegan. I found that if I told people, instead, that it was a zero carb or keto-diet, then they usually found that more acceptable. The word "carnivore" seems to cause a knee-jerk reaction, so feel free to avoid using it.

I've also described it to some people as "an elimination diet to determine allergies." No one wants to mess with someone trying to figure out allergies. People usually back down when that is the "diet" being described. Again, you don't have to use the word "carnivore" when describing the diet.

And finally, it just doesn't get any better than letting results speak for themselves. When most people witness dramatic changes in your health or weight loss, they'll want to know how you did it. For the rest, the permanent naysayer types, being in freaking amazing shape has a funny way of making them STFU.

Plan Ahead to Avoid Breaking the Bank

The carnivore diet can seem more expensive if you're coming from a diet of cheap, refined carbohydrates. There are many ways to decrease the cost however, which I address in Chapter 8.

Practice Cooking

Figure out your favorite meats and practice preparing them. When I started the carnivore diet, I was pretty good at making a steak, but not every one of them came out perfectly. Within the first month, I learned about the reverse-sear method which was helpful for thick cuts of steak (learn how to use this method in Chapter 14).

I also struggled with making ground beef patties. My usual method was in a skillet with fat splattering all over the place and only being able to cook a few at a time. I learned how to broil them on a baking tray so I could make 8 at a time. That was great because I could easily fortify my family this way. Also, I could cook patties in advance if I made a lot at one time like this.

Speaking of advance cooking, that's another tip. Make larger portions of carnivore foods that are ready to grab and eat (or quickly reheat). It's easy with methods like broiling a bunch of ground meat patties or using a slow cooker (or Instant Pot pressure cooker) for roasts. (See Chapter 14 for recipes.)

As mentioned earlier, Dr. Shawn Baker often repeats the mantra "eat meat like it's your job." Once I heard that, I realized I had not been doing it. Eating more beef helped my fatigue during the transition keto-flu. It also helped avoid losing too much weight, which I did the first few days from not eating enough.

Over time, my appetite increased naturally and everything leveled out, including the ability to maintain a great shape and weight. A carnivore dieter will quickly learn what satisfies him or her the most (beef for some, lot of cheese for others). It's also common to eat fewer meals and make them bigger. Some people like eating only once a day. I don't usually do that. I've found that two meals a day is perfect for me. I certainly don't feel the craving or desire to snack between these two meals because I'm usually full enough, for hours. But, if you're hungry for a snack? Snack on meat.

I'll address boredom, though I don't see it as an issue. It never was for me. I think in the beginning, having a lot of variety with animal products and by-products ensured no boredom. There were so many choices. I was excited to eat bacon and eggs in the morning, a bunch of chicken drumsticks for lunch, and big slab of beef for dinner. Some days I had fish instead of chicken. Some days I had ground beef and other days I had ribeye (both beef, but such different experiences). So many options, zero boredom.

Repetition is the mother of skill," says Tony Robbins. It really applies to the carnivore diet. Whether a carnivore dieter finds happiness in eating only ribeyes and water or a bit more diversity by rotating a few different animal products repeatedly, the ease of this schedule makes it easy. Once you settle into a routine, you'll find your groove and things will just click. The beginning is for experimentation though, so have fun with it. Go crazy.

Stay Hydrated

This is not only important but it's a good hack during cravings. I keep a big jug of water on my counter and my goal is to have it finished by the end of the day (not drinking too far into the evening, or I'll have to pee in the middle of the night). When I go into the kitchen, this water is the first thing I see, which reminds me to drink. Staying hydrated this way helps me drink less coffee, stay satiated, and feel well.

Eat Fatty Cuts of Meat

I can't emphasize this enough. One of the easiest ways to transition into a carnivore diet is being sure to eat enough fat. It can take getting used to for some people, and for others it's a joy (it was a joy for me). The fat has nutrition and adds to satiety. I think it plays a big role in helping keep cravings at bay, too.

This means I gladly eat the skin on chicken, I happily embrace the fat on pork, and I choose fatty beef or add fat to it. For example, I opt for ground beef that is 20% fat. If I can't find that, I buy the highest fat content I can find, and I add fat to the meal via butter, ghee, lard, and/or cheese.

Another tiny little hack I have for eating fatty ground beef is I bake my ground beef in something that saves all the fat and juices that cook out (a baking tray or a baking dish). Then, I serve my ground beef in a bowl, I pour the juices and fat over the ground beef, and I eat it with a spoon. This ensures I get lots of juicy fat with each bite.

Salt Foods to Improve Electrolyte Balance and Deliciousness

I don't track my salt intake, and I'm not afraid of salt, specifically sea salt. It makes my food taste delicious, and I feel great. I salt all of my animal meats, especially my bone broth.

I've heard of people in the transition phase possibly experiencing electrolyte imbalance resulting in cramps. I'm not a doctor and not prescribing anything here, and I didn't experience this. Some people find that with salt on the food and drinking water, it's helped. Some people might supplement during the transition phase.

Here's some useful information from ZeroCarbZen.com:

"When you first go on a low-to-no carb diet, you lose a lot of excess fluid from your cells. As this fluid gets flushed out from your body, it carries electrolytes with it. … Many folks who experience muscle cramps when they first begin a Zero Carb diet have found that both extra salt (containing both sodium and chloride) and extra magnesium can help to prevent muscle cramps during the transition process. However, increasing these three electrolytes is not universally helpful, and it is my opinion that potassium is often the electrolyte that most needs to be supplemented.

"The RDA for potassium is about 5,000 mg per day. It takes about 3 lbs of fresh meat to meet this requirement. Whether the RDAs are the same for people following an all meat diet is certainly open to debate, but I offer it here for reference."

Keep a Food Journal

I found that journaling my daily food intake and experiences was useful in the transition phase.

Journaling inspired me. It also allowed me to track everything and make adjustments. I think journaling food intake is one of the most important carnivore diet transition hacks. You'll see excerpts from my carnivore food journal in Chapter 15.

Take Before-and-After Pictures

Stop what you're doing, right now, and go take a picture of your upper body. Although I didn't take before and after pictures, I wish I had. (I forgot actually, otherwise I would have.) I love seeing when other people do it. It's a great testimonial and motivator for others. It's a super way to stay motivated yourself.

Take Advantage of the Carnivore Community for Inspiration

I found following different carnivore dieters on Twitter and Instagram really fun and useful. It put rocket fuel in my tank for excitement, getting ideas, and learning more.

If you spend enough time in these communities, you might find yourself getting caught up in drinking the Kool-aid, which can clearly help, but it can also have its drawbacks. If for some reason this diet doesn't work for someone, the community can create a placebo-type effect. You might ignore negative factors, which is not good. I'm extra cautious of this because of my experience with vegan communities back when I ate a vegan diet. I saw success stories and felt surely that they were applying to me. When I started having problems with my health, there was a long period where I wasn't open-minded enough to question if they were from the diet.

The important thing to remember is to always listen to your own body and intuition. It's not a religion, it's food. Always remember that.

Personally, I would still find a lot of value in these groups, reading articles about other people doing this, and following people doing it on social media. Just do it with your eyes wide open and listening to your body.

Online Support Groups and Forums

- The Carnivore Training System online health coaching by Dr. Shawn Baker
- Dr. Shawn Baker on Twitter: @SBakerMD
- The nEqualsMany experiment started by Dr. Shawn Baker
- The World Carnivore Tribe Facebook group
- The Zero Carb Health Facebook group
- The Principia Carnivora Facebook group
- The Zero Carb subreddit forum

Eat a Flex-Meal or Have a Flex-Day

A flex-meal or flex-day just means allowing yourself a meal or day when you go off the carnivore diet and eat whatever you want. You could do it once a week, for instance.

This option is to add flexibility without stress. You have allowances for some plants, if the occasion arises. I don't recommend doing a flex-anything however, if it tends to start a cascade of carbohydrate cravings, as it can with some people.

Some would call this a "cheat" meal, but that's a negative word and could set someone up for failure. Language is important for success. I call it a flex-meal or a flex-day and it's more relaxed. It's not cheating, it's a deliberate part of the plan (if it's part of your plan). There's no stress or guilt.

During my first 60+ days on the carnivore diet, I did not want or need any flex-meals/days. However, I had to end the strict carnivore eating plan because we embarked on a long-term journey traveling the world. It took me a while to regain my carnivore footing in foreign lands, but after a couple of months, I found myself able to easily get back on the carnivore diet. I learned where to find the best sources of affordable meat in our new location. After that, I was able to stay strict with it again. No flex-meals/days needed.

That was, until we traveled again. Travel days were difficult since I had to eat out, especially in unfamiliar cities. So, I created a "travel day carnivore meal plan" (see chapter 11) that gives me ideas for staying carnivore on travel days when it's hard. However, I remind myself that I'm comfortable partaking in a flex-meal/day on travel day if it's needed. Sure I would prefer to stay carnivore on a travel day, but things can happen, and giving myself flexibility relaxes me.

If you are going to have a flex-meal, try eating something that's not too far from the diet, such as fruit or a sandwich made with traditional sourdough surrounding plenty of meat and cheese, or maybe some dark chocolate. While most of these aren't parts of a meat-only diet, they're not as bad as something with overly processed and refined carbohydrates.

If you decide you do want to include in your strategy a flex-meal/day, schedule it as a regular event, say every Saturday or every other Sunday. Then, if you choose to not partake, that's fine. Wait until the next designated time. I wouldn't just assume that if I skip, say Sunday, I could move it to Monday or it might create chaos for me. Having a set schedule will ensure no snafus and help keep the diet on track.

CHAPTER 7: HOW TO FEED YOUR NON-CARNIVORE FAMILY

I'm the chef of the house. My family doesn't eat exclusively carnivore like I do. They love eating meat with me, but my husband loves his microbrew beer, the occasional carbs, and sampling local fare as we travel. As a result, I still have some vegetable chopping to do, but it's less than it was in my pre-carnivore life. I used to be famous in my family for daily, elaborate gourmet salads. Shortly after going carnivore, my husband noticed something was up when I served his delicious steak with nothing but one little sad-looking raw carrot. My husband looked up and said, "I see you went all out on the veggies, honey." I laughed out loud... he was right. He has since come to call such low-effort vegetable sides as "the passive-aggressive carrot" and "phoned-in veggies."

I do still serve my family vegetables, but I'm more selective and I serve mostly non-sweet fruits (in the technical botanical sense, meaning it has seeds, such as red bell peppers). I don't often bother with dark leafy greens or broccoli; I'm no longer convinced they're necessary. My family instead eats more things like bell peppers, tomatoes, cucumbers, celery, fennel, tubers, and occasional sweet fruits. They also eat traditionally fermented sourdough bread (sourdough's bacterial fermentation makes it much healthier than yeast-leavened bread). They enjoy high-fat dairy and dark chocolate. When we go out, they get what they want (healthy, but more traditional), and I get what I want (keeping it carnivore).

Therefore, my family's meal prep, though not as quick as my carnivore meals, doesn't take me too much extra time. Shopping, again, is longer since I'm not just heading straight to the meat department, but it's not bad.

I don't feel the need for tons of variety on the plate. I don't favor heavy and dark greens. I opt for more protein and healthy fats for us all. I now tell my kid to EAT YOUR MEAT instead of preaching "eat your vegetables." Not surprisingly, now that she eats more beef, she asks for dessert less often.

CHAPTER 8: HOW MUCH DOES IT COST TO EAT A CARNIVORE DIET?

The cost of eating a carnivore diet depends on a few factors.

Consider first, however, that non-carnivores spend a lot of money on things like lattes, supplements, superfoods, and medications, to name a few.

Does this describe you? If so, what if you stopped buying them? How much money would you save? Enough to pay for loading up on beef at every meal?

I mention medications because those can be expensive, and I've heard about a lot of people who reduce or stop taking their medications when they eat a keto or carnivore diet (check with your doctor!). And, also, check out the website MeatHeals.com for many testimonials about that.

Many people also eat a lot of meals at restaurants, which usually costs more money than eating at home.

Then, there's the cost of the meat. Cost-per-ounce will vary a lot based on the source (sardines vs. halibut, chicken vs. beef), and the cut (ground beef vs. filet mignon).

And if you want to opt for only grass-fed or organic products, then naturally it'll cost more money. Is this necessary? It's personal preference. As described earlier, according to Dr. Shawn Baker, most conventionally raised cattle indeed spend a lot of time eating grass and only get confined and fed corn during the last phase before slaughter. Some people don't like the taste of grass-fed beef and prefer the sweeter meat of a corn-finished one anyway.

Besides, then there are the people who think that corn-finished beef is better for you, because it's typically fattier than a grass-fed animal, and fat is very good for you. That's food for thought.

But I'd say that most people think grass-fed is more nutritious from higher vitamin levels and lower omega-6 fatty acid levels. I counter that with this idea: eating a carnivore diet alone is nutrient dense and avoids other foods typically very high in omega-6 fatty acids, and so it's probably not a concern.

Furthermore, there are other animal products much higher in omega-6 fatty acids, such as chicken and pork, but you don't hear about that as often. I think the carnivore diet, which has no seed oils (those are high in omega-6 fatty acids) will automatically be more nutritious when looking at omega 3 to omega 6 ratios. If for any reason I feel like I should add more omega 3s to my diet, I could reduce the poultry and pork for more beef. Also, I can simply bust out a can of sardines or mackerel (or cook some salmon).

When my goal is frugality I get some things pasture-raised and others not. If I'm buying anything pasture-raised or grass-fed it's usually high-fat dairy and eggs (the costs are reasonable). These items also aren't a large part of my diet, which makes it easier to spend a bit more for higher quality. I also only choose wild-caught fish, which is expensive. Therefore, I don't buy wild-caught fish very often. An exception is canned sardines and mackerel, which are great, frugal options).

To recap:

1. Decide whether you want to spend the extra money on grass-fed animal products or not.
2. See if there are other things you can cut out of your life to pay for the extra meat.

How I Eat a Frugal Carnivore Diet

If I'm not careful, the cost of eating meat can really add up. But with some planning, it's manageable.

I can eat a no-frills carnivore diet for about $4 a day. I weigh 123 pounds. If I were a bigger person, such as a 200-pound man who works out regularly, I estimate it would cost $6 - $7 per day, no frills (ground beef, sardines, etc.), and $10 - $15 per day eating sale-priced steak. More, if you eat grass-fed beef or pasture-raised poultry. (For more on saving money, see my book, *The Frugal Carnivore Diet: How I Eat a Carnivore Diet for $4 a Day*.)

MyGroceryDeals.com

If I'm spending more than $7 per day because I want steaks, the first thing I do when I'm in the USA is use this awesome coupon site. This is the best way to search all the local stores for sales on meat, especially ribeye steaks. I can find ribeye steaks for $6 a pound (this would not keep me at a $7/day). Ground beef is much cheaper. In fact, I can often find grass-fed ground beef for a great price, too. Price is dependent on the cut of the beef, so consider that.

Mailers and Flyers

I always check the sales flyers that are mailed to me from the grocery stores. It's a great way to plan ahead.

Use a Local Butcher

If you're lucky enough to have a local butcher, it's a great way to go for fresh meat. They will tailor the cuts to your preferences. Also, if you buy enough or become a regular customer, you can often negotiate better prices.

Local Farmers and Ranchers

You can usually find these folks at local farmer's markets selling their animal products. Some of them will have CSA (community supported agriculture) weekly delivery options, too. My experience is that these tend to be grass-fed products and so they're still on the higher side for prices, but lower than buying from a store. These people can be open to negotiation, too. If they don't have a CSA, maybe work out a weekly schedule and work out a lower price, too.

Discount Stores

Investigate local discount stores, such as Costco (USA), Tesco (UK), and Aldi (Europe). These can be great places to find animal products for much less. When we sold everything to travel the world, it was

Tesco that enabled me to get back to my carnivore diet in the United Kingdom. I found great prices there. The same happened for me in France with Aldi, but unfortunately the selection was limited and usually sold out. If that's the case, wherever you shop, ask what days they receive meat shipments and plan your shopping around that.

Buy Part of a Cow

Yes, really. Don't worry, it doesn't look like those carcasses Rocky punches in the freezer. The meat comes in neat little frozen packages. When we lived in the USA, we had a separate standalone freezer. I used to buy an ⅛ of cow a couple times a year. Buying part of cow, whether corn-finished or grass-finished, can significantly reduce prices. You can find this option at a butcher, with a rancher, or online.

Buy a FoodSaver

One of the best kitchen inventions, next to the Instant Pot, is the FoodSaver. It's a great way to eat a frugal carnivore diet. Remember my tip of using MyGroceryDeals.com? I would go to the store with the cheapest ribeye steaks. I'd buy 10 to 20 if I could (sometimes the store has limits, which I got around by bringing my husband and/or mom with me). I'd take the steaks home and package them using the FoodSaver by putting two in a bag at a time. Then, I'd stack them in the freezer.

Buy an Extra Freezer

Whether buying an ⅛ of a cow, loading up at Costco, or stocking up when you find a great sale or coupon, you need space for the meat. Having an extra freezer really helps you multiply the value of sales. Be mindful of the extra electricity cost however, if you live in a warm climate and/or have expensive electricity in your area. In particular, you don't want to be paying for electricity if your freezer is sitting mostly empty.

Group Purchase in Bulk

If you don't have an extra freezer, or if you just want to split the cost of a bulk purchase, go in on it with one or two family members or friends.

CHAPTER 9: HOLIDAYS ON THE CARNIVORE DIET

How do I navigate the holidays while eating a carnivore diet? I have some tips to share, but in the end it's all about:

- Planning
- Treating oneself with extra ribeyes
- Setting expectations with family and friends
- Maybe taking the holidays off with Flex-Meals/Days

Planning

I start my planning early when it comes to holidays. That means communicating with family and friends. I have no problem telling my family that I'm eating a certain way. I'm not shy about it. They're also really used to it by now. I send an email in advance telling everyone how I'm eating and that I plan to stick to it. If I feel compelled, I tell them how great I feel, how my allergy problems were improved, weight was lost, whatever… I basically list the benefits I experienced and how I want to keep it that way. Then, I ask them for their support (people like to help, they want to be on the team). Finally, I tell them I'm happy to bring my own ribeye or extra serving of meat if needed. I never want to put the host out for my diet. I tell them I'll be following my same diet through the holidays. If I'm happy and feeling awesome on the diet, then a holiday is simply just another day.

For people on regular weight-loss diets, feasting holidays like Thanksgiving and Christmas can be brutal, sometimes adding pounds in days that took months to lose. Not so for carnivores! Fortunately for us, these same holidays usually come with plenty of meat on the table. Woohoo! Feel like splurging? Fine, splurge by eating more meat!

Still, the fancy dessert table, or that stuffing that only mom knows how to make, might beckon you from across the table. I combat this by making sure my carnivore meal included my favorite meats: ribeye steak and bacon. Once I filled my belly with those, I'm a happy camper, feeling better than everyone else sitting around the table in their food-comas. Meanwhile, I could throw on some running shoes and take a jog, or do some squats and pushups, because I'd feel like such a strong bad-ass.

Sometimes there are holiday gatherings for the office (or other parties), where things like appetizers make the rounds. In those cases I'd simply fill up on beef before going. I'm so satisfied with carnivore foods that I'd likely be content for hours. But, just in case, I'd stick an Epic beef bar or beef stick in my purse (Epic bars aren't cheap protein, but they're great in a pinch). I'd also drink coffee (regular or decaf) at these events if I needed a beverage in my hand and water wasn't cutting it. Sparkling mineral water is a great option, too.

Lastly, if you really want to have mom's childhood-memory-inducing stuffing, then consider implementing a flex-meal/day, and be smart about the size of your ONE portion (the flex is to let you be flexible, not foolish).

Warning: If you're not already used to flexing and it's not a regular part of your carnivore diet, be aware that you might feel ill having plants or foods processed in ways you don't normally cook. You might also start a sugar craving cascade. Do so at your own risk. But I think it's totally doable (provided you don't really have bad allergies to plants). In fact, if I did it, I'd probably end up feeling crappy and sluggish and it'd inspire me more to get right back to meat-only, starting with those wonderful 10pm Thanksgiving night fridge-raiding leftovers snacks... but only the meat.

Lastly, if you decide to do a flex-day/meal during a feast, load your first plate with meat only. Maybe your second plate, too. Then when you sample the stuffing or pumpkin pie, you'll at least be full enough to be disciplined about taking only small portions.

CHAPTER 10: THREE APPROACHES TO THE CARNIVORE DIET

Here are some ways to approach the carnivore diet, or a diet that is meat-heavy. With all three options, some people keep coffee and tea in the diet, as a drug and not a food, and many others gravitate to just water. Therefore, I won't mention coffee in these options listed below specifically, just know some people include coffee and tea.

Option 1 Carnivore

Animal meat, animal fat, water. Simple and popular.

Option 2 Carnivore

Animal meat, animal fat, animal by-products (high-fat dairy), water.

Option 3 Mostly Carnivore

Animal meat, animal fat, animal by-products (high-fat dairy), water, occasional plants. This is not a full carnivore diet, though it might still be a keto diet, depending on the frequency of the plants eaten.

For example, perhaps once a week, add a small handful of berries or a small portion of a tuber. Maybe a bit of honey in the diet.

Or, maybe it's every other week.

Or, maybe it's on the night of the full moon every month.

You decide.

Our pre-agricultural ancestors didn't have access to fruits, tubers, or honey on a daily basis, year round. It was most likely seasonal, depending on where they lived. If you wanted to mimic that diet, you'd include plenty of space between consuming those items. (Bearing in mind that today's cultivars are only distant relatives of their ancestors. They've changed a lot; we haven't.)

Some people do well on this diet and the carbohydrates don't affect their cravings. Others want to stay away from all carbohydrates because it induces cravings. Yet others stay away due to allergies to the plants. It all depends on the individual.

Unknown Allergies to Plants

After having eaten a carnivore diet for six months, I ate a bell pepper one day, when I was staying in rural France, as my meat options were a bit limited way out in the country. I was shocked to feel my lip start tingling.

On a separate occasion, I ate an apple and my tongue started tingling. The interesting thing is that I had felt these sensations before, back in my plant-eating days, but I just shrugged them off because they weren't painful or too severe. I didn't even think to associate them with food allergies. They're fruits, after all... and healthy, *right?*

Not necessarily. Having that experience after eating carnivore for months, it really stuck out to me, because it never happens to me on a carnivore diet. I realized it was not normal. My tongue and lips shouldn't feel that way after eating food. I've since learned that, if I have a few bites of either of those things once in a while, no big deal. But if I eat a whole one, I have a reaction. Um... no thanks!

CHAPTER 11: TRAVELING ON THE CARNIVORE DIET

Traveling while eating a carnivore diet can be done with a few tips.

Here are good travel day carnivore food ideas and tips whether traveling by train, plane, car, internationally or domestically.

Big Dinner the Night Before

Although it's not always easy to plan, I'll often eat a big meal of beef the night before traveling. Then, I fast (with water and/or coffee) as long as I can the next day (the travel day). I like the simplicity of this idea because I don't have to pack food or think about it much.

(Fasting may sound extreme, but "intermittent fasting" — a little fasting each day — can be extremely effective for losing weight. See my book, *Carnivore Diet Intermittent Fasting* to learn how these two dietary hacks work so well together.)

Bone Broth in a Thermos

I love carrying bone broth with me on a travel day because it's warming and satiating. I always ensure some of the chicken fat, beef fat, or pork fat is in the broth. If I feel like my broth doesn't have enough fat, then sometimes I'll add butter to it.

Before leaving for the day, I'll warm the broth on the stove, stir in some butter and sea salt (if needed), and transfer the drink to a thermos. I might also add a protein powder like collagen to give me more "food" if I won't have access to quality food where I'll be traveling. It helps me stay full a bit longer having more protein. I recommend the collagen from Andrew Lessman (made from tilapia fish) and Upgraded Self (from beef).

Another awesome option is to make my Ground Beef Patty Chicken Broth Soup (see recipe, Chapter 14) and put that in a thermos. It'll stay hot for hours in a good thermos and makes for a super nourishing and satisfying meal. Keep in mind TSA restrictions on liquids if you're headed to the airport.

Buttered Coffee Protein Shake
(Large size, with or without protein powder, hot or cold.)

If I'm opting for coffee, I sometimes amp it up with calories, fat, and protein, by mixing protein powder and butter in it. It's delicious and satisfying.

Here are variations I go through (the coffee can be regular, decaf, or a mix). I'll make this in the morning before I leave (using a blender, ideally) and pour it into a huge thermos:

- Hot Coffee + Butter

- Hot Coffee + Butter + Protein powder
- Hot Coffee + Butter + Protein powder + Ice
- Hot Coffee + Butter + Ice

Blending the hot coffee with the butter is important (and protein powder if applicable) so the butter gets dispersed.

Then, if opting for ice, I'll either pour it over a bunch of ice or I'll blend in the ice after the coffee, butter, (and protein) are blended.

I'll drink this on my way to the airport and finish it before going through security. Then, I'll take the empty cup to refill with coffee (possibly cream) after going through security.

Protein Powder and Water

Again with the protein powder. I'm not a huge fan of having any reliance on these because, of course, I'd rather eat meat. However, travel days can wreck a great carnivore diet. I have no desire to be sad on a travel day because I'm hungry and don't have meat available.

I remember one trip where we were at the airport early and there was only one restaurant open that had meat. It was in the form of shredded beef and it had been cooked with vegetable oils (which I didn't want). I knew I was getting on a long plane ride. I had a few beef sticks with me, but honestly, I can only eat so many of those before I feel ick. But, I didn't want beef cooked with vegetable oils (they promote inflammation).

So, I went to the coffee shop and bought a large decaf coffee and loaded it with heavy cream. It was a learning lesson that I need to plan better. I realized that if I'd had a protein shake with fat in it, I'd have been much more satiated. A protein shake like that, along with a couple beef sticks, now that would be great.

So, if I'm not drinking coffee or don't want multiple cups of coffee with protein powder, I'll bring protein powder with me, and I'll mix it with bottled water (could be plain collagen or plain whey - something I can easily shake with water.) Of course, having a thermos of this already mixed up is a solid plan, too. Then, pack extra protein powder for later once that pre-mixed drink is consumed.

Coffee/Tea with Heavy Cream

Coffee and tea is quite satisfying to me and curbs my appetite, so I'll take advantage of this and use it as a travel hack. Adding heavy cream can keep me going for a couple of hours, at least. I love cappuccinos, too, if whole milk is available.

Water or Sparkling water

Drinking plenty of water, although not exciting, can keep my hunger at bay for awhile, especially if I'm watching a great show on my iPad or listening to a good podcast. Sparkling water, in particular, adds to the satiety by filling your stomach with a comfortable amount of CO_2 gas. Starbucks usually sells San Pellegrino sparkling mineral water, and there are usually Starbucks in airports and many on the road when on road trips.

Hard-Boiled Eggs

These can really make a great difference on a travel day. The protein makes my belly happy. I'll cook a dozen of them the night before a travel day. I may or may not leave the shells on, it depends on the travel day.

On travel day, I pack them in a Ziploc bag and I bring a second bag for the shells, if they're not peeled. I also pack a little baggie or container of sea salt (which I always travel with anyway). I make 12 eggs so I can have 6 and my husband can have 6. My young daughter doesn't love the yolks in hard-boiled eggs, so usually nibbles on the whites of some of mine.

The shelf life on these is not great since they're not refrigerated. I don't carry them with me all day. I eat them usually within a few hours of packing them. However, when I'm road-tripping in a car, I always pack a cooler, in which case these eggs can stay cold for the day and I have the flexibility of eating them whenever I get hungry.

Cured Meats/Beef Sticks

I always have these packed in my purse, backpack, and luggage. Cured meats like salami or ham also have a short unrefrigerated shelf life, like the eggs, above. So I eat them early on in the travel day (think airplane travel) unless I have a cooler (think car road trip).

Beef sticks/Jerky, like Epic bars etc are packaged to last and those I can pack and eat any time of the day.

Cheese

I sometimes pack a hunk of cheese on a travel day and follow the same protocol as eggs and cured meats in that I don't let it stay unrefrigerated for more than a few hours. My husband especially loves the cheese. It's satisfying for me, as even just a few bites can buy me some time until I can get my hands on some beef.

Canned Fish

Canned fish such as sardines and mackerel with a pull-top lid are very portable and can have a shelf life of more than five years. I like to pack them, but we're limited in where we can eat it due to the smell and potential mess. At a gas station, no problem. In an airplane, not a chance. So, while it's a great carnivore diet food to keep me filled up (frugal, too), I have to be choosy when I eat it.

However, I always pack a few cans in my luggage because there are many times that we land at our destination and don't get a chance for good food until later in the night. Between airport transfers, lack of restaurants with beef patties, and getting to our destination and then trying to find a place to eat... I bring cans of fish for this exact reason. I can tear into one right when I get to our location.

(Sardines are so amazing in so many ways that I could write a whole book about them. In fact, I have: *The Sardine Solution: How and Why to Eat the World's Most Badass Source of Protein*. Not a fan of these little amazing fishies? You just might become a convert by the time you're finished!)

Strategic Distraction

If I'm in one of those positions where I'm fasting or drinking just water or coffee and I'm feeling like I might end up getting hungry, I'll deliberately distract myself. I listen to a podcast of something inspiring to me (or entertaining), or I watch a favorite movie or TV show series. Or games, if you prefer. Lastly, sleep always works if that's possible.

Tips for Airports

When I'm at an airport, I first seek out the available food options. Sometimes there are fast food joints with all beef patties, which is ideal. Other times there aren't!

We were in a terminal one time where they had a burger place but it was a fancy restaurant where a patty would've cost me over $10. No thanks, unless of course I was totally starving. In that event, I would've tried to have them substitute butter, bacon, and cheese instead of the bun, pickles, and lettuce.

If I can't find any beef, I'll do some of the things I listed above regarding water or coffee with cream (again, *coffee ain't carnivore*).

But, guess what? Some Starbucks sell sous vide eggs! Some of these have cheese and meat in them. One time I loaded up on eight of them. I've also bought their sandwiches and picked out the meat between them. It's neither satisfying nor cheap, but it got me through a travel day sticking to carnivore foods.

I always take advantage of walking and push ups on travel days to stay healthy, strong, motivated, and to keep my workout momentum going... otherwise it's very easy for travel to disrupt your consistency. I'll walk while waiting at the airport (or train station) to distract me and get some steps in before sitting on a long flight (or train ride). I also find a quiet corner to do some push ups. People might glance over, but I don't care and they quickly lose interest. I always feel strong and better about myself when I do these things.

Things I Pack When Traveling

What I pack depends on whether I am going in a plane, train, or car. It depends on where I'm staying once I arrive too, and the climate. However, here are things I consider bringing:

Flying

Options are very limited when you're flying. You can't carry much volume in carry-on in the cabin (and no knife, of course), and I prefer not to check luggage whenever possible. And if I do check luggage, I avoid including anything expensive. Just a small knife sharpener and a thin cutting "board" (it's just a thin sheet of plastic that could be rolled, but I lay it flat in my suitcase so it doesn't curl) can turn a shitty AirBnB with a dull knife and no cutting board into a serviceable kitchen for a couple of days.

As noted below, I also always bring a meat thermometer if I'll be checking luggage. (The stabby part might not make it through security and I don't want to risk trying.)

Road trips

If we have the space in the vehicle, I will try to get away with packing lots of different things.

Instant Pot

Instant Pots are fantastic, versatile pressure cookers that can save you a ton of time and generally make your life better. I can plug it into hotel rooms or in apartments. It's a favorite way to cook hard "boiled" eggs, certain cuts of meat, and bone broths. They make a mini-version that I haven't tried yet, but it would make it that much easier to pack.

If I'm packing for a stay in a hotel room, I usually also pack a cutting board for setting my meat on, along with anything else I might normally use. The key is to imagine yourself going through the steps of cooking and eating. What would you use? Thinking this way, I'd also need tongs. Keep in mind that if you're cooking in a hotel room you'll need cutlery and plates. Sometimes the hotel has these things and other times they don't. Plan accordingly. Sometimes I take the plates from our camping gear and pack those. They're lightweight, durable, and pack tightly.

A hotel is different from renting an apartment, condo, or house through AirBnB. Those places usually have kitchen things like knives, tongs, cutting boards, skillets, etc. I always check with the host in advance. Pro tip: always pack a small knife sharpener. AirBnB's are often stocked with the lowest possible quality gear, and a sharpener will make even a crappy knife work for cutting your meat.

Slow cooker

Although I prefer my Instant Pot to a slow cooker, I brought my slow cooker on a few trips before I owned an Instant Pot. I didn't use the slow cooker in hotel rooms, but I did at AirBnB's and once when I visited my brother for two weeks. (Note: the Instant Pot actually has a slow cooker function, but I find it useless because my unit always got too hot.)

Cooler

Having a cooler in a car is a must for me. I can pack hard-cooked eggs, cold cuts, cheese, butter, etc. On ice, these items can last a couple days.

Meat Thermometer

Meat thermometers are the key to perfectly cooked meat, every time, as well as safety against foodborne illness. I pack this no matter where I'm going, although, as mentioned above, I haven't tried to get it through airport security, so I'm not sure if they would require me to check it.

Salt

I always pack my own sea salt so I have some whenever I need it. I don't pack a lot because once I get somewhere I can buy it if I'll be there long enough to buy groceries. However, if it takes a day to get to a grocery store once I get somewhere, I like to have some on hand. Sometimes I just fancy a pinch of it when I'm feeling hungry and I can't get my hands on any food.

Planning Ahead

Before I go on a trip, I *always* plan ahead regarding stores and restaurants. I look for frugal stores like Costco, Tesco, Aldi, etc. I also pay attention to the local restaurants. As you'll see in a moment, we cook most of our meals, so my focus is always on stores rather than restaurants.

I also keep my eye out for fast food restaurants with all-beef patties while on the road and once we've arrived at our destination. We don't make these staples though, because I'm the only one in the family who eats just the patties (or patties with cheese). If my husband and daughter are with me, they'll eat the buns, mustard, and ketchup, which is fine once in a while, but not for regular eating.

Renting Apartments: My Favorite Travel Hack

By making sure we're in an apartment instead of a hotel room, I can always cook. There's usually cooking equipment there, and I don't have to bring mine, or not as much. I'm no stranger to cooking with a hot plate and skillet in a hotel room not designed for it... I've used the tiny bathroom sink to wash a large skillet and blender containers. And I'd prefer not to. (It's a bit silly and fun – the first time. But it gets old fast.)

The point is that I go to the extreme to ensure I'm eating the way I want. I don't just let my diet go to shit because I'm traveling. I don't use that as an excuse. With some basic planning, it can be quite easy for me to stay on a carnivore diet while traveling.

Lastly, I'll say this. If I'm traveling and all the cards dealt to me just aren't making it convenient, easy, frugal, or feasible to realistically stay on a carnivore diet, I'll just make it as carnivore as I can. Then, I'll supplement with plant foods, mostly fruits and vegetables. I'm not convinced I need to be carnivore every day for the rest of my life. I like it for now, though, and I aim to keep it going when possible. If I'm traveling and I need to have some plants, they're not going to kill me.

CHAPTER 12: CARNIVORE MEAL PLANS

See Food Journal (Chapter 15) for Options I Tried

You'll see that in the beginning of my food journey with a carnivore diet I kept coffee and tea in it. I had a variety of meats and included full-fat dairy. Over time, like most people, I gravitated to a carnivore diet with mostly beef.

1 to 3 Meals a Day

On a carnivore diet, eating becomes less of a to-do because everything is simplified. And satisfaction is high, so people have fewer (or zero) cravings for anything other than simple animal products (and maybe coffee, because caffeine is an addictive drug after all).

As a result, some people eat only one huge meal a day. That could mean having 2 to 5 pounds of beef *in one sitting*, depending on the person and his or her exercise intensity. I don't expect a more sedentary 5-foot woman to eat 5 pounds of beef, but it could happen to a 6-foot+ man who is training hard.

More often, I see people eat two meals a day, but it's perfectly fine to eat three meals a day. The important thing is to follow your appetite. That's one reason Dr. Shawn Baker says coffee can be a problem, because it can curb your appetite in the morning and then you might eat less in the day. (On the other hand, my husband likes morning coffee specifically for this reason.)

Personally, I drink coffee most mornings, and, yes, it curbs my appetite in the morning. Which is fine, because I don't always want to dive into meat in the early morning. Some mornings, I replace my coffee with bone broth, which is satisfying and delicious.

If you drink coffee but would like to quit, or reduce your intake, one approach is to try starting the day with a big glass of water and then dive right into some meat or eggs. It might help break your coffee addiction. Again, bone broth is another great option.

Remember, people on a carnivore diet *eat until they are full*. That's really *the* key of the carnivore diet. They let their appetite guide them. They never need to worry about eating too much.

The cool thing about carnivore meal plans is that they're all just a rotation of a small number of foods with plenty of combination options. So, the repetition is intrinsic and one of the brilliant aspects of the diet. This repetition is what makes the diet so easy, decision-making-fatigue-free, and helps ensure fewer cravings.

Here are the most common meals I have while on a carnivore diet. Which one I choose on any given day is mostly determined by where I happen to be staying on that day.

Breakfast Ideas

- Water or coffee (heavy cream optional), 3 to 5 eggs cooked in butter

- Water or coffee, 3 eggs cooked in butter, cheese
- Water, coffee, leftover meat from the dinner before
- Water, meat I cook (steak) for breakfast (i.e., not leftovers)
- Water, bone broth
- Water, bone broth, 3 eggs whisked into the bone broth while it's heating on stove which cooks the eggs
- Water, bone broth as above with 2 eggs, plus grated cheese stirred in
- Water only, if fasting until lunch or dinner, because I ate a huge meal the night before

Lunch Ideas
- Anything from the breakfast ideas list above
- Water, 2 cans sardines or mackerel, plus something from the breakfast ideas
- Water, cheese, salami (I wouldn't have this daily)
- Water, bacon, bone broth

Dinner Ideas
- Anything from the breakfast or lunch lists above
- Beef: roast, patties, meatloaf, meatballs, steak
- Chicken on the bone
- Non-canned fish (salmon, cod, shrimp, etc.)

CHAPTER 13: CARNIVORE DIET SHOPPING LIST

Let's go shopping! My list is usually: beef, chicken, canned fish, eggs, cheese, salami, bacon, butter. It's small by nature, which makes shopping easy. Get in and get out.

I love the times when I walk straight to the butcher counter, buy a bunch of ribeyes and head straight to the check-out. Done. It's during those shopping visits that I want one of Dr. Shawn Baker's "Carnivore AF" t-shirts.

But… a full carnivore diet shopping list, well you can have plenty of options as shown below.

Animal & Animal By-Product Options

- Beef & bison (ground, chuck roast, steak… any cut)
- Lamb/mutton & goat
- Elk & venison
- Poultry: Chicken (whole or in pieces), turkey, duck, wild fowl (quail, pheasant, etc.)
- Pork (bacon, pork shoulder, ham, etc.)
- Rabbit
- Fish (canned mackerel in water, canned sardines in water, canned wild-caught sockeye salmon, whole fillet wild-caught salmon)
- Shellfish, shrimp/crawfish, octopus/squid
- Organ meats: Liver, heart, tongue
- Dairy (heavy cream, butter, ghee, cheese)
- Eggs
- Sausage (bratwurst, salami, etc.) & jerky
- Bone broth

CHAPTER 14: CARNIVORE RECIPES

Note on Yields

Unlike my other recipe books, for these carnivore recipes, I'm intentionally not featuring yields. I don't know how many servings a recipe will provide since we're all a bit different in how much meat we choose to eat.

As a carnivore dieter, I look at the amount of meat in a recipe and then estimate how many meals I'll get from it. And, honestly, sometimes I eat a pound of meat in a sitting, sometimes more and sometimes less. It just depends.

Use these recipes as training for preparation of carnivore diet foods. My goal is to show some different ways to cook animal products. From there, you can decide whether to double the recipes, or cut them in half, etc., based on how many people you're serving or how many meals you'd like to create for yourself.

General Protein Cooking Tips

Here are some of the most helpful things I learned in culinary school, where I took a course in classical cooking after years of eating a vegan diet, and having no idea how to cook meat.

Salt Your Steak or Fish Just Before Searing

It's good to make sure you've pat the protein dry with paper towel, too, to ensure a good crust from the sear (otherwise it could cause the protein to steam instead of getting a good sear). So… pat dry, season with salt, and then sear right away.

Eggs Keep Ground Beef Moist

I like having egg added to most of my ground beef dishes (think meatloaf and meatballs), because it stays more tender and moist. I add 1 egg per pound of ground beef.

Make Sure Your Skillet Is Hot!

Get that pan hot before searing the protein. Also, once the meat is in the pan for searing, don't fucking touch it. Let it get its sear on, uninterrupted, which for me is usually something like this:

- Beef: 1 to 3 minutes per side, depending on the cut
- Fish: 1 to 2 minutes per side
- Chicken breast (with skin): 5 to 7 minutes per side

Just remember, the protein should easily come off the pan when it's ready to flip with a spatula. If it's stuck to the pan, let it cook longer. And, as chef likes to remind us, "Use your head and common sense. If you're searing the protein and it looks like the pan is too hot, then lower the heat." See? Common sense.

At this point, you either serve the protein because it's cooked to temperature, or you might need to finish it in the oven. The following oven temperatures are good rules of thumb though you can adjust them as needed:

- Red meats (375 degrees F)
- Fish/Pork (350 degrees F)
- Chicken (325 degrees F).

The time needed to finish cooking depends on the thickness of the protein, too. Remember when I said I always travel with a meat thermometer? Now you know why. I use an "instant read" digital thermometer ($25-100), which is one of the best kitchen gadget investments I've ever made.

After removing beef or poultry from the oven, "rest" it about 1/3 of the cooking time. So, if it takes 30 minutes to cook your meat, it should rest about 10 minutes. It's not a hard and fast rule, but a nice guideline.

What the Duck?

By the way, duck is considered a red meat. (Who knew?) You may never cook duck in your life, but if you do, know that duck meat is treated by many chefs differently than what they do for other poultry.

Thermoworks, the company that makes my favorite Instant Read Thermometer that I travel the world with, has this to say about duck:

"Sure duck is technically 'poultry', but when it comes to cooking this aquatic fowl, traditional cooking techniques just won't do … consider the duck, which much like the turkey has differing degrees of dark meat. Though duck meat in general is much darker, closer to lamb or beef, with its myoglobin a rich purple color.

"That being said, the breast is still lighter and should only be heated to 135°F to avoid drying out the meat. The thighs and legs on the other hand should be heated to 165°F to help break down connective tissue and produce a more tender dish.

"Most may see 135°F and think that that's much too low for a poultry dish, and generally you would be correct. The USDA recommends 165°F internal temperature for all poultry. But because duck is not a common carrier of salmonella and its meat is more akin to lamb or beef, Hank Shaw, author and chef, says, 'Rare-to-medium is the mantra' when it comes to duck breast. And, with medium rare ranging from 130 to 135°F according to the USDA, this fits perfectly with the cooking of this less common bird."

Sous Vide Eye of the Round

The <u>sous vide</u> (pronounced "soo veed") is also called a *water oven*, which is similar to a slow cooker, but the temperature is tightly controlled and the food is cooked in a vacuum sealed bag fully submerged in water. This allows you to cook any food, such as a steak (or any cut of meat, including beef tongue, chicken, turkey, fish and more), to tender, juicy perfection, every single time. The meat cooks all the way through, to the exact temperature you want, and it will never overcook. Awesome, right?

The sous vide makes life easy, because it means I can put the steak in my sous vide to cook, early in the morning, and not worry about taking it out to sear until I'm ready at lunch or dinner, or heck the next day, and it won't dry out. This means I don't have to "time" my steaks to be done at a certain time. For guidance, there are plenty of websites (and apps) featuring recommended cooking times when using a sous vide.

Equally important is that using a sous vide allows me to cook much less expensive cuts of meat to "tenderloin tender" which saves a lot of money. I can also make huge batches of bone broth with the Sous Vide Supreme (see my blog post here for directions).

You'll see later in this recipe section that I also love using my slow cooker and Instant Pot (pressure cooker) for cooking tough cuts of meat because they make those cuts tender like the sous vide. The sous vide won't overcook the meat, which can happen with a slow cooker or Instant Pot.

I personally use and highly recommend the Sous Vide Supreme Water Oven. Here are a couple of tips for using it on meat:

- Fill the sous vide with warm water to get it heated to the target temperature faster.
- Sear the meat after removing it from the vacuum-sealed pouch for a more attractive presentation (about 45 to 60 seconds per side in a hot skillet with some animal fat). Some people pre-sear the meat before putting it in the sous vide. That said, searing is totally optional.

How to Make Perfect Eye of the Round in a Sous Vide

- 1 (3 to 5 pound) eye of the round steak
- sea salt
- ghee or lard

1. Fill the sous vide with warm water, and set it to 136 degrees F (or your preferred end temperature).
2. Once the sous vide has reached temperature, get your eye of the round from the refrigerator.
3. Put it in a FoodSaver bag with a spoonful of ghee or lard.
4. Vacuum seal the bag and put it inside the sous vide for 24 to 32 hours.
5. Take it out, pat it dry with a paper towel.
6. Heat a skillet hot with ghee, lard, or butter.
7. Season the eye of the round with sea salt.
8. Sear it on all sides (about a minute each side).

Sous Vide Steak

- 1 to 4 steak(s)
- sea salt
- ghee or lard

1. Fill the sous vide with warm tap water.
2. Turn it on to the desired cooking temperature. For my steaks, I usually set it at 134 degrees F.
3. Once the sous vide is heated, get the meat from your refrigerator.
4. Season the meat with salt.*
5. Get FoodSaver bags (1 for each steak), and fold the top of each bag over a bit to keep food from touching the part of the bag that needs to be sealed.
6. Place one steak in each bag. Unfold the bags back to original position after the food is in the bags before sealing.
7. Vacuum seal (I use a FoodSaver to suck out the air and seal the bags.)
8. Put the sealed steaks into the sous vide and cook for the desired time. I usually let my ribeye or New York strip steaks cook 4 to 8 hours, depending on my schedule.
9. Take the vacuum sealed bags out of the sous vide after cooking. Cut open and take the meat out (it will look kind of grayish, which is normal).
10. Dry the meat by patting it with a paper towel.
11. Get a skillet hot. Add some butter, ghee, or lard, if desired. Sear both sides of the steak(s) (while basting with the butter if getting fancy), for 45 to 60 seconds per side.

* Seasoning with salt before putting it in the sous vide, or after searing in the skillet, is personal preference. If it's meat that I'm cooking for longer than 10 hours, I tend to season it *after* cooking.

Reverse-Sear Oven to Skillet Steak

This is a brilliant way to get perfect cooking of any size steak when you don't have a sous vide.

The reverse-sear method will take a bit longer than just cooking it in a skillet only, but with a bit of planning, it's mostly hands-free. The idea is that slowly cooking it in the oven ensures even cooking. Once you take it out, a quick sear gives flavor and color without risk of overcooking.

- steak (any size or cut)
- sea salt
- ghee, butter, or lard (for searing)

1. Season the steak with salt.
2. Nestle a cooling rack inside a baking tray. Place the steak on the rack nestled inside the baking tray.
3. Turn the oven on to 275 degrees F. Put the steak inside. *If it's a thinner steak, I cook it in the oven for 20-25 minutes. If it's a thick ribeye I cook it for 40-45 minutes. I like a final internal temperature of my steak (after searing) to be ~125 degrees, so I keep the steaks in the oven for those aforementioned lengths of time, depending on the thickness of steak. The time also depends on how cold the steak was, coming from the refrigerator. Essentially, I keep them cooking in the oven until the internal temperature of the steak in the oven reaches about 110-115 degrees F.*
4. Heat a skillet to medium-high. Add a bit of fat (butter, ghee, or lard).
5. Sear the steak on each side for about a minute.

Broiling Patties

This is the easiest and cleanest way to make multiple burger patties, and clean up after is a snap.

- ground beef*
- sea salt
- cheese, if desired

1. Line a large baking tray with aluminum foil.

2. Generously season the beef with salt. On average, I use ½ to 1 teaspoon per pound of beef. It depends on taste and the coarseness of the salt.

3. Create patties from the beef: Roll each one into a ball and place it onto the aluminum foil-lined tray. Then smash them into patties, pretty thin to cook faster.

4. Place the rack in the oven so the burgers will be about 3 to 5 inches from the top burner and turn on the broiler.

5. Place the tray of patties on the top rack and cook for 3 to 4 minutes. Flip them and cook another 3 to 4 minutes, until desired temperature is reached. If using cheese, place the cheese on top of each patty and return under the broiler for about 30 seconds.

* I like to let my ground beef sit for about a half hour (or a bit longer), after taking it out of the refrigerator, to get closer to room temperature for better cooking.

Cheesy Meatloaf

This recipe is fun because when you cut into the meatloaf, melted cheese oozes out. It's the simple things, right?

- 2 pounds ground beef
- ¾ to 1 teaspoon sea salt, more to taste
- 2 eggs
- 5 to 7 ounces cheese, in slices, chunks, or grated

1. Preheat the oven to 350 degrees F.
2. Whisk the salt and eggs in a large bowl.
3. Add the beef.
4. Briefly mix it all together so the egg and salt is dispersed throughout the meat.
5. Press half of the mixture into a meatloaf baking dish.
6. Place the cheese as a middle layer.
7. Press the remaining half of beef on top of the cheese, as the top layer of the meatloaf.
8. Bake for about 50 minutes, depending on the internal temperature you prefer.

Meat "Brownies" (With or Without Cheese)

No, these don't have chocolate in them. I call these "brownies" because I bake them in a 9x13-inch baking dish, and when I cut and serve them as squares, the shape reminds me of brownies. My family prefers cheese on them. I prefer them without cheese. Therefore, I put cheese on one half for them and the other half is without cheese for me. Everyone is happy.

- 2 pounds ground beef
- ¾ to 1 teaspoon sea salt, more to taste
- 2 eggs
- optional: sliced or grated cheese

1. Preheat the oven to 350 degrees F.
2. Whisk the salt and eggs in a large bowl.
3. Add the beef.
4. Briefly mix it all together so the egg and salt is evenly dispersed throughout the meat.
5. Press the mixture into a 9x13-inch baking dish.
6. Bake for 20 to 25 minutes, depending on the internal temperature you prefer. If you are planning to add cheese, add the cheese during the last 5 minutes of cooking so it melts nicely.

Simple Meatloaf

An easy way to make my entire day's food is to make this in the morning, and eat it all throughout the day. Cook once and eat twice (or three times). This recipe has the same ingredients as the Meat "Brownies" (without cheese) but it's in a meatloaf shape.

- 2 pounds ground beef
- ¾ to 1 teaspoon sea salt, more to taste
- 2 eggs

1. Preheat the oven to 350 degrees F.
2. Whisk the salt and eggs in a large bowl.
3. Add the beef.
4. Briefly mix it all together so the egg and salt is evenly dispersed throughout the meat.
5. Press the mixture into a meatloaf baking dish.
6. Bake for about 50 minutes, depending on the internal temperature you prefer.

Easy Broiled Parmesan Meatballs

If you make the meatballs using about 2 tablespoons each of the beef mixture, you'll get about 30 meatballs.

- 2 pounds ground beef
- 2 eggs, lightly whisked
- ½ to ¾ teaspoon sea salt, more to taste (keep in mind that cheese is salty, too)
- 1 cup freshly grated parmesan cheese

1. In a large bowl, combine the whisked eggs, salt, and cheese.
2. Add the beef and mix it all together so the egg, salt, and cheese is evenly dispersed throughout the meat.
3. Form meatballs using a tablespoon (I use an ice cream scoop), 2 tablespoons per meatball.
4. Place each meatball onto a baking tray with a lip to catch the juices and fat. Broil them for 7 to 10 minutes, depending on the internal temperature you prefer.
5. Serve the meatballs with their meat fat and juices drizzled on top.

Beef Chuck Roast — Oven Braise & Pressure Cooker Recipes

There s not much that I like better than a big-ass chuck roast that s tender and full of flavor. It warms my soul to enjoy those big spoonfuls of shredded beef, juices, and broth.

Pro-tip: All roasts should be brought to room temperature before cooking, to ensure even cooking throughout. Seasoning is also essential, so be sure to season your roast with plenty of salt before cooking.

Oven Braise Directions

This recipe is for making a chuck roast in the oven under low temperature. This recipe takes time in the oven, so plan accordingly. Even better, make this a day in advance of eating it. The flavors will intensify. Just reheat on the stove before serving.

- 1 (2 to 6 pounds) chuck roast, bone-in preferably
- salt
- 3 cups bone broth (or water)

1. Preheat the oven to 200 degrees F.
2. Cut the roast into quarters. Season it generously with salt.
3. Put the seasoned beef and the broth in a Dutch oven (or similar pot with lid) into the oven. For now, though, do not use the lid. Cook until the meat and broth reach 120 degrees F (about two hours).
4. Cover the pot. Increase the temperature of the oven to 250 degrees F and cook it until the meat is 180 degrees F (another 3-4 hours)
5. Test for tenderness. As the saying goes, "the meat should tremble when the fork approaches." If it' s not tender, cook longer, testing in 20 to 30 minute increments.

Instant Pot Directions

I love making chuck roast in the <u>Instant Pot</u>, a popular electric pressure cooker. I loved mine so much that, when we left to travel the world, I seriously tried to find a way to pack my beloved appliance in my suitcase. In the end, I opted for traveling backpack-style and, obviously, that wasn't going to work. The Instant Pot makes tough cuts of meat tender and succulent in record time.

- 1 (2 to 4 pounds) chuck roast, bone-in preferably
- sea salt
- 1 cup bone broth, unsalted

1. Quarter the chuck roast and season it generously with salt.
2. Pour the bone broth into the Instant Pot. Add the beef.
3. Secure the lid. Cook under HIGH pressure for 55 to 75 minutes. (Time will depend on the weight of the meat, as well as whether the meat was closer to room temperature before cooking or straight from

the refrigerator. Experiment to find what time works best for you. Once you figure it out, write down the details for future use.)

4. Let the Instant Pot naturally release the pressure.

5. The beef should basically ⊠tremble as the forks approach it⊠ for shredding. If it s not tender, cook under HIGH pressure for another 5 to 10 minutes, and try again, with no need to naturally release pressure. You can quick release it at that point.

Whole Chicken Instant Pot

The <u>Instant Pot</u> delivers yet another awesome meal, quickly. The chicken comes out nice and tender. Leftovers, if there are any, can be stored in the refrigerator for quick eating and bones can be used for bone broth.

- 1 (3 to 5 pounds) whole chicken
- 1 cup water
- sea salt

1. Put the water and the steamer rack into the Instant Pot.
2. Generously season the chicken inside and out.
3. Put the chicken in the Instant Pot. Secure the lid.
4. Cook on HIGH pressure for 15 to 25 minutes (*5 minutes per pound* of chicken). Let the Instant Pot release its pressure naturally.
5. Take the chicken out and set aside to cool a bit until you can handle it.
6. Pull the meat off the bone. Shred or chop the chicken.
7. Save the bones for broth (see recipe later in this chapter)

Spatchcock-Roasted Chicken

A recent conversation I had with my dad, the retired chef:

Dad: "You did *what* to the chicken?"

Me: "I spatchcocked it."

Dad: "What the hell is that?"

Me: "I simply cut out the backbone and spread the damn thing open like a book! It's a chicken hack to make it cook faster. Didn't you know?"

It's never too late to learn a new trick in the kitchen.

- 1 (3 to 5 pounds) whole chicken
- sea salt
- melted ghee, butter, or lard

1. Preheat the oven to 375 degrees F.
2. Spatchcock the bird: With a sharp knife, kitchen shears, or even garden shears (my preference), remove the backbone by cutting up along each side of the backbone and removing it. Save the backbone for making chicken broth.
3. Flip the chicken over, and open it like a book. Spread it open and firmly press down on the chicken with both hands to flatten it. (There are many videos on YouTube.)
4. Generously season both sides of the bird with sea salt.
5. Lay the bird on a baking tray, skin side up. Drizzle some animal fat on top.
6. Roast the bird for 45 to 60 minutes or until deepest part of the thigh reads 165 degrees F on a meat thermometer.
7. Transfer to a cutting board and let it rest for 10 to 15 minutes.
8. Carve and enjoy.

Cast Iron Skillet Oven-Roasted Chicken

- 1 (3 to 5 pound) chicken, whole
- sea salt
- ghee, butter, or lard

1. Preheat the oven to 350 degrees F.
2. Generously season the inside and outside of the chicken with salt.
3. Heat some animal fat in the skillet over medium-high heat until it's hot.
4. Put the chicken, breast-side down, in the skillet and cook until it's golden (about 5 minutes).
5. Carefully flip the bird onto it's back and brown for another 5 minutes. Sometimes I add a bit more fat to the skillet, if needed. To help with the flipping, I insert a long-handled wooden spoon to help lift the chicken.
6. Carefully transfer the skillet and chicken to the oven and cook for about 60 minutes, until a thermometer in the deepest part of the thigh reaches 165 degrees F. Time will vary based on the size of the chicken.
7. Remove the skillet and the chicken from the oven. Allow it to rest for up to 15 minutes before carving.
8. Save the bones for bone broth.

Roasted Chicken Drumsticks

- chicken drumsticks
- sea salt
- melted butter, ghee, or lard

1. Preheat the oven to 350 degrees F.
2. Spread the drumsticks out on a baking tray, roasting pan, or baking dish. I like to have a bit of space between them when possible, for better airflow in crisping the skin.
3. Season both sides of the drumsticks generously with salt.
4. Drizzle some melted butter, ghee, or lard on top of them.
5. Roast the drumsticks for 35 to 40 minutes, flipping them halfway at 20 minutes. Cook until the internal temperature, close to the bone, reaches 165 degrees F using a meat thermometer.

Chicken Bone Broth

I'm going to share how I quickly make chicken bone broth. I don't let it cook for 12 hours if I don't have the time. It's often just a couple of hours. I usually make it from the bones from drumsticks, since that's my favorite way to cook chicken (it's so easy).

I wrote <u>a whole book about making bone broth</u>, including beef bone broth (as well as using a sous vide or the oven). For this discussion, I'll focus on chicken bone broth because it's my favorite. (For options with a slow cooker or <u>Instant Pot</u>, see the bottom of this recipe.)

- bones from chicken
- cold water

1. Place the bones into a pot.
2. Fill with enough cold water to just about cover the bones.
3. Turn the heat to high and keep an eye on it. You want it to just barely get to a boil. Then, turn the heat down to simmer.
4. Let it cook for up to 12 hours (I usually do 2 to 4 hours if I'm in a hurry). If you let it go a long time, you need to keep an eye on the water level as you'll likely need to add some throughout the cooking time.
5. Scoop out the bones and throw them away.
6. Pour the broth through a strainer (if desired, for clear broth) into a big bowl or a large glass Pyrex liquid measuring cup. *I often just skip the strainer and do my best to keep some of the extra bits out that I couldn't get when scooping out the bones.*
7. Once it's cooled a bit, transfer to glass mason jars. If you can, put the lids on them (if they're not too hot). To speed up the cooling at this point so you can put them in the refrigerator, put them in a cold water bath. I don't advise using ice or the glass might break from the sudden temperature change.
8. Store in the refrigerator for up to 5 days. When it's cooled in the refrigerator, the fat will rise to the top. If there is not a super thick disc of fat, I keep it there and melt it while it's heating when I cook it. Therefore, I drink it in the broth. However, if it's a really thick puck of fat, I'll cut some of it off and leave some in the broth. The part I cut off, I'll dry with a paper towel and cook with it. If I'm not using it right away, I'll store it in the refrigerator and use within a few days.
9. To serve the broth, warm the amount you want on the stove and season with sea salt. I like plenty of sea salt in my broth.

Alternatively, you can cook the bones in an Instant Pot or slow cooker:

Instant Pot

Put the bones in the Instant Pot and add enough water to just about reach the top of the bones. Secure the lid. Cook under HIGH pressure for 60 minutes. Quick release or natural release, it's up to you. Let it cool a bit, strain out the bones, and follow the remaining instructions, above.

Slow Cooker

Put the bones in the slow cooker. Add enough water to just about cover the bones. Turn the slow cooker on HIGH and put on the lid. Let it cook for about 12 hours. Strain out the bones and follow the remaining steps, above.

Bone Broth Egg Drop Soup

- 2 cups bone broth
- 2 eggs, lightly whisked
- sea salt, to taste

1. Heat the broth on the stove to a simmer.
2. Slowly pour the eggs into the soup and stir to create a cooked ribbon of eggs.
3. Once the eggs are cooked to your liking, pour the soup into a big mug or a bowl.
4. Taste and season with salt.

Bacon Egg Soup

- 2 cups bone broth
- 2 eggs, lightly whisked
- 2 to 4 strips of *cooked* bacon, chopped (see recipe for Slow No Splatter Oven-Baked Bacon, later in this chapter)
- sea salt, to taste

1. Heat the broth on the stove to a simmer.
2. Slowly pour the eggs into the soup and stir to create a cooked ribbon of eggs.
3. Once the eggs are cooked to your liking, pour the soup into a big mug or a bowl.
4. Stir in the cooked bacon.
5. Taste and season with salt.

Bone Broth Egg Cheesy Soup

This is a hearty version of bone broth.

- 2 cups bone broth
- 2 eggs, lightly whisked
- 2 to 4 tablespoons freshly grated parmesan cheese
- sea salt, to taste

1. Heat the broth on the stove to a simmer.
2. Slowly pour the whisked eggs into the soup, and stir to create a cooked ribbon of eggs.
3. Once the eggs are cooked to your liking, pour the soup into a big mug or a bowl.
4. Add the cheese and stir to mix.
5. Taste and season with salt.

Burger Patty Chicken Broth Soup

Here's a nice twist on leftover ground beef patties (or meatballs, etc), if you have chicken broth in the refrigerator. Make a comforting and filling soup mixing the two.

- Cooked ground beef leftovers (patties, meatballs, etc)
- Chicken bone broth

1. Put the two items into a soup pot on the stove, and cook until warmed through, breaking up the chunks of meat.

Baked Salmon

- 1 to 4 pieces (4 to 6 oz each) wild-caught salmon, skin on
- melted ghee, butter, or bacon fat
- sea salt

1. Preheat the oven 375 degrees F.
2. Place the salmon skin-side down on a baking tray or in a baking dish.
3. Season the fish with salt. Drizzle a bit of melted animal fat on it.
4. Bake it for 20 to 30 minutes, until desired doneness is achieved (time varies based on thickness of the fish). I cook my salmon until the internal temperature of the thickest part reaches 120 degrees F using a meat thermometer. (For farmed salmon, it's recommended to cook to 125 degrees F.)
5. Optional, serve with melted butter (or bacon fat).

Pan-Roasted Salmon

- 1 to 3 pieces (4 to 6 oz each) wild-caught salmon, skin on
- melted ghee, butter, or bacon fat
- sea salt

1. Preheat the oven to 350 degrees F.
2. Pat the salmon dry with paper towel.
3. Heat some animal fat in an oven-safe skillet and get it very hot(!) – but not smoking hot. Season the meat side with salt.
4. Put the salmon pieces into the pan, meat-side down. Make sure they're not overcrowded. Cook for 1 to 2 minutes. You're getting a sear on it, and it should release from the pan easily with a spatula once it's ready, provided your pan was hot enough at the start. (Some chefs start skin-side down, but this is personal preference.)
5. Flip the salmon and cook the other side (the skin side) for 1 to 2 minutes.
6. Transfer the skillet to the oven and let it cook until it reaches the desired temperature, which, for me, is 5 to 8 minutes, depending on thickness of the salmon (I like the internal temperature of the thickest part of the salmon to be 120 degrees F. For farmed salmon, it's recommended to cook to 125 degrees F).
7. Optional, serve with melted butter (or bacon fat).

Simply Sautéed Shrimp

Shrimp is easy to make, though shrimp alone doesn't satisfy me for a meal. I like to serve it with beef for surf-n-turf.

- wild-caught shrimp, (fresh or frozen/thawed), peeled and deveined
- ghee, butter, bacon fat

1. Rinse the shrimp. Pat dry with a paper towel.
2. Get a skillet warming over medium-high heat with some animal fat melting in it.
3. Once the skillet is warmed through and getting hot, add the shrimp and cook for 1 to 3 minutes each side, depending on the size. Then, stir frequently until they're done. They're done when they've turned opaque and pink in color.
4. Season with salt, to taste.

Shredded Pork (Instant Pot)

I could eat this for days on end. Think ahead and make a big batch so you can do the same.

- 1 (2 to 4 pounds) pork shoulder/butt roast, bone-in preferably
- medium-coarse sea salt*
- 1 cup water

* Judy Rodger's rule for salt: Use about ¾ to 1 teaspoon of medium-coarse salt for every 1 pound of meat.

1. Leave the pork whole, or cut the roast in half, thirds, or quarters. Smaller pieces cook faster.
2. Sprinkle the salt evenly over the pork.
3. Add the water to the Instant Pot.
4. Place the seasoned pork in the Instant Pot. Cover and secure the lid.
5. Set the Instant Pot to HIGH pressure for 90 minutes, if the pork is whole (and on the heavier side), or halved. For thirds or smaller pieces, cook 70 minutes. If it's a smaller-weighted roast that's also quartered, like two pounds, try cooking for 60 minutes.
6. Let the Instant Pot slow release naturally.
7. Check that the pork is fork-tender. If it's not, cook the pork under HIGH pressure for another 5-10 minutes. Quick release the pressure this time.
8. Transfer the pork into a large bowl and shred the pork.
9. Taste the cooking liquid remaining in the pot. Adjust the seasoning with water or salt if needed. Add as much of the cooking liquid as desired to the shredded pork.

Slow No-Splatter Oven-Baked Bacon

I don't like standing over a stove cooking bacon in a skillet while it splatters everywhere. Not to mention, most skillets can't fit my whole package of bacon in one batch, which means I stand there longer. Using the oven solves all of my problems. I don't stand around and there's no splattering.

- 1 package sliced bacon

1. Set the oven to 300 degrees F.
2. Place the bacon strips on a baking tray with lipped edges to prevent the fat from pouring off. Alternatively, you can use a large baking dish. I like that the bacon cooks in its fat instead of setting it up to drip through a cooling rack.
3. Place the tray or dish in the oven (it doesn't have to be preheated to start).
4. Cook for up to 60 minutes, or until desired doneness is achieved.

Skillet Cooked Veal Cutlet

- veal cutlet
- ghee or lard
- sea salt

1. Flatten the veal so that it's even, if needed.
2. Get a pan hot(!) with a bit of animal fat, but not quite smoking hot.
3. Season the veal with salt, when the pan is hot and ready.
4. Put the veal in the pan, lay it down while facing the pan away from you to prevent hot fat splashing on you. Cook for 1 minute each side. Then, cook longer, if desired, to reach preferred temperature of doneness.

Hard-Boiled Eggs — Stove and Instant Pot

Traditional Hard-Boiled Eggs

Hard-boiled eggs are great to have in the refrigerator at all times. They make for the quickest breakfast or mid-night snack ever (even faster than my dear sardines).

- water
- 12 eggs (or fewer)

1. Get a pan and put cold water in it.
2. Add the eggs (in their shells).
3. Bring the water to a boil. Turn the heat off. Take the pot off the burner.
4. Cover the pot and let them sit in the hot water for 8 to 9 minutes (you can experiment and see if you like the yolk's hardness at 7, 8, or 9 minutes - it depends on your preference).
5. While the eggs are cooking, prepare an ice bath (a bowl filled with half ice and half water).
6. Using tongs, immediately transfer the eggs into the ice bath to stop their residual cooking.

Instant Pot Hard-Cooked Eggs

My favorite way to cook hard "boiled" eggs is with the Instant Pot, cooking them under pressure. There is one reason: IT'S EASY. It makes taking off the shells easier than any other method (there's science involved - it has to do with quick heating and fast cooking). They come off quickly and in big chunks, leaving the egg white intact because the shell isn't sticking to the egg. It's such a popular way to cook eggs that the pressure cooker is dubbed the "magic egg machine."

- 1 cup water
- 12 eggs (or fewer)

1. Pour the water into the Instant Pot. Add the steamer rack.

2. Gently put the 12 eggs inside (you can cook fewer if you want). Secure the lid.
3. Cook on LOW pressure for 3 to 5 minutes depending on desired doneness (I prefer 3 to 4 minutes).
4. While they're cooking, get an ice bath ready (large bowl with half water and half ice).
5. Once the Instant Pot is done cooking… quick release the pressure.
6. Transfer the eggs to the ice bath with tongs.
7. After letting the eggs cool a few minutes, you can easily peel off the shells.

CHAPTER 15: MY CARNIVORE DIET FOOD JOURNAL

In this chapter, I've included an excerpt of my food journal from when I first went carnivore, around January of 2018.

I love journaling because it inspires me and also allows me to troubleshoot. I didn't include the whole journal here because that would be a lot of reading. It's just my quick notes and reflections I had, plus the foods I ate for the day.

At the time of this writing, I've gone on the diet twice, only because I was forced to quit temporarily by circumstances, which I describe after the journal excerpt.

Food Journal - My First Time Eating the Carnivore Diet

Day 1

I went cold-Turkey essentially, though it was a gradual shift to carnivore since my meatloaf had some non-carnivore things in it (my mom was cooking that day). I also had MCT oil. I was testing the waters without much planning, and eating what was on hand. I didn't do any activity other than living life and running errands. I felt fine and satiated with excitement about trying this.

- Sardines
- Meatloaf (had breadcrumbs and green onions, ketchup)
- Meatloaf (again)
- Can tuna with MCT oil drizzled on top

Day 2

Overall felt awesome and empowered. Spent a lot of time sitting because I was reading more on carnivore eating from others. Had a touch of a headache but it went away. Excited to try this carnivore eating experiment for 30 days as I read more. I think I will cut out MCT oils and olive oils and also reduce coffee and tea going forward.

- 4 eggs cooked in ghee with cheese
- Black coffee
- Bulletproof decaf coffee
- Shrimp with butter and salt
- Green tea x 2
- Chicken sausages
- Buttered coffee

Day 3

I woke with a sinus headache and went straight for the Americano but made the coffee a bit weaker. I slept well last night and again, I woke bright eyed and bushy-tailed. Later in the day, I felt a bit anxious but my blood pressure was good. Headache went away after I took 1 ibuprofen. I don't normally resort quickly to ibuprofen for pain, but decided I had too much to do today and didn't want to do it with pain. Also, I could be experiencing "Keto flu" as described by others. It's minor for me personally. Two hours later, feeling better. Felt better rest of day. Feel totally satiated and have zero desire for anything other than animal foods.

- 2 x Americanos (brewed weakly)
- 5 eggs cooked in ghee
- Chicken sausage leftovers
- Decaf coffee with butter and ghee
- 1.5 pieces bacon
- 5 oz beef patty cooked in bacon fat
- 2 scallops
- 5 oz beef patty cooked in ghee
- 2 oz beef patty cooked in ghee
- 2 cubes cheese

Day 4

Woke again bright eyed and bushy-tailed. Still have small headache seems like sinus and pollen counts are high so maybe that's the cause (or it's still "Keto-flu"). I'm not hungry though coffee curbs appetite. Finally had eggs at 11am. Wasn't hungry again until 4pm. I didn't have much choice in food because of traveling so I opted for buttered coffee to increase calories and satiation. Headache was only mild on and off today. Took half an aspirin mid-day and it's stayed gone since. Relieved at the ease of food prep... Loving that and loving NOT being hungry and loving NOT being obsessed with food thoughts all day.

- Americano
- 4 whole eggs + 1 yolk gently scrambled
- Green tea
- Can sardines
- 2 oz cheese
- Decaf coffee with butter
- 6-8 oz ground beef
- Decaf buttered coffee

Day 5

Woke up feeling great again. Had coffee because I think I'm just going to slowly wean off it. It ended up really curbing my appetite though and I wasn't hungry until 11am, when I decided I should just eat so I could fortify myself. After eating the eggs, I was full all day. I ate oysters, again just to get something in my stomach. I felt a bit anxious today because we have a lot going on in our lives at the moment (all good and exciting stuff nonetheless still a lot to process) but I also felt happy and strong. Had a tiny altitude headache like I usually get after coming home to Carefree where there's a tiny bit of elevation compared to Sun City West. Bottom line: today I had basically no appetite. Was cold later in the day (winter), and felt I should probably eat more, so I had three fried eggs.

- Black coffee
- 4 whole eggs + 1 yolk gently scrambled
- 5 smoked oysters
- Ground beef and ground offal with cheese on top
- Buttered coffee
- 3 fried eggs in ghee

Day 6

Feel great and have been busy. Hardly any hunger. Super satiated and have to remind myself to eat. Food's role in my life has changed. I just eat to fortify and that's it. Simple.

- Black coffee
- 4 eggs cooked in ghee
- 6 oz ground beef patties
- 5 chicken drumsticks, roasted
- Decaf buttered coffee

Day 7

Again, I woke refreshed. I decided to get calories immediately by having butter in my coffee. I'm just not very hungry, and I think I'm losing too much weight. I feel mostly excellent, but again feeling a bit anxious because we have so much going on with moving to Europe. It's all manageable though with meditation.

I'm very busy and don't think to eat. For dinner I wasn't super hungry but thought I better eat. I've lost 3-4 pounds in one week on this carnivore diet, and thought I should eat more.

For dinner, I ate an 8-ounce (before cooking) patty, cooked in ghee. I felt fortified. I'm in bed feeling very relaxed now. I had a busy day with things getting checked off my to-do list. I have good energy through the day, but that could be because I'm busy. Or the diet?

- Coffee buttered
- 2 raw egg yolks and 1 can sardines
- 2 raw egg yolks (I put them in a shot glass and chug them down)
- Green tea
- 3 chicken drumsticks, roasted
- 2 x buttered decaf coffee (one with teaspoon MCT oil)
- 1 chicken drumstick
- 8 oz beef patty
- 1 oz raw cheese

Day 8

Ok so it's been a whole week. Interesting. I think I went through some fatigue a couple of days but overall felt excellent in spirit and mind. Loved the lack of thought about food. I read last night that if people feel tired or weak they need to remember that on this plan you "eat meat like it's your job" - in the beginning especially. I haven't been doing that. It's not easy and I aim to increase my calories today.

I also started my cycle so was in the pre-cycle phase this last week and that could have had an impact on energy levels. I sometimes get tired a couple of days in the week ahead of my cycle.

I'm not sure what to make of the sleeping. I sleep very well, dream, etc, but I'm waking earlier than normal. Does my body not require as much sleep? Today I woke before 5am. I went to sleep last night around 10:00 or 10:30 pm. Maybe that's good sleep and all is well or is this style of carnivorous eating messing with my sleep negatively? Or, maybe positively.

Maybe it's that I'm not using my digestion as much, and I learned long ago that digestion is a big energy user. Maybe my body doesn't have as much to do at night and so I wake earlier. Or, again, I just have lots to do before we move and that's taking center stage.

- Buttered coffee with tiny drizzle MCT oil (really for extra calories, as I don't think I'll keep MCT in my diet once my current bottle is used up)
- 3 raw egg yolks (these are easy to chug down)
- Mint tea
- 8 oz beef patty
- 4 oz patty
- Chicken (small: thigh, leg, breast)

Day 9

I woke again with ease. I'm guessing this is par for the course by now, and I'll stop mentioning it, unless it changes. I haven't exercised much and I'm ready to start. I have had consistently energetic days lately, and I want to combat any stress by working out.

I'm still drinking coffee and not sure when I'll cut that out… it is half decaf though so I'm not needing full caffeine.

I'm lean and happy with the constant flat belly!

Feeling great throughout the day today. Not hungry, as usual, but eating anyway. Bought some whipping cream to add calories and diversity.

- Black coffee
- 6 raw egg yolks
- Buttered decaf
- 2 oz ground beef
- 4 oz steak
- 3 oz salmon
- Decaf with cream
- Patty with cheese

Day 10

Another fine morning. Felt great yesterday and strong, though I've still been forgetting to exercise with my long list of to-dos. I do meditate though – there's always time for that.

- Black coffee
- 3 raw egg yolks
- Ribeye steak
- Coffee with heavy cream
- Beef patty with melted cheese
- Coffee with heavy cream

Day 11

I woke up early again and today I started doing a little bit extra movement. I did some rebounding and a little bit of strength training. I'm going to add some more later today.

Later: I never got around to the exercise "later" because I ended up running errands that took me longer than expected. Didn't have a food plan so I ate some cheese at mom's – just a couple cubes and had some tea. When hungry and in a bind, cheese totally kicks ass. It satiates with just a couple of bites.

- Black coffee
- 6 raw egg yolks

- Mint tea
- 3-4 oz beef patty with cheese
- Decaf with heavy cream
- 1-2 oz cheese
- 4 oz cod with a little butter
- 2 oz salmon
- Decaf with heavy cream

Day 12

Still doing this. I want to have more offal but I just don't like it. I started my day with hot water in place of coffee thinking the coffee curbs my appetite too much. I need to eat more on some days. I feel fine otherwise.

(Whoops. Looks like I forgot to record food.)

Day 13

- Egg yolks
- Coffee with heavy cream and collagen powder
- Ground beef with cheese
- Baked fish: cod

Day 14

Feeling good and normal. Busy.

- Coffee black
- Ground beef
- Decaf coffee with heavy cream and collagen powder
- Green tea
- Decaf coffee with heavy cream and collagen powder
- Ground beef with tiny squirts of mustard and hot sauce
- Decaf with heavy cream

Day 15

Woke after 7 hours of good sleep. I've stopped losing weight and it's stabilized nicely. I feel crazy doing this, but I want to stick it out and see what happens after a month.

- Black coffee
- 6 raw egg yolks
- Decaf coffee with butter and collagen powder
- Beef patty with cheese

- Beef patty with cheese

Day 16

I seem to be ready to rock-and-roll after 7 hours of sleep. I used to want/need to get 8 to 9 hours, but I'm ready to wake after 7 hours these days.

- Black coffee ☕
- Buttered coffee with collagen powder (using this up because I have it)
- 5 raw egg yolks
- 3 slices cheese
- 5 smoked oysters
- Buttered coffee with collagen powder
- Salmon sockeye canned
- Hot dogs (all beef)
- Beef patty with cheese

Day 17

All is very well. I wish I were testing my strength more. I'll try more movement and exercise tomorrow.

- Black coffee
- Decaf buttered collagen coffee
- Hibiscus tea 3 oz
- Steak
- Cheese
- Cheese beef patties

Day 18

- Coffee
- Ghee + collagen blended Coffee
- 8 oz steak
- 1 sardine
- Cheese beef patty
- 6 oz steak
- Buttered decaf x 2

Day 19

Skin is amazing. It looks so pretty, the color and clarity. Energy solid. Emotions great. I have consistently felt super. I like the buttered coffee in the morning because I'm not really hungry in the morning, and feel like I want something, but not ready to dive into eggs or meat. This is a nice light intro. I poop everyday, sometimes twice. It's simply smaller amounts because it's not bulked with fiber.

- Green tea
- Coffee with butter and collagen powder blended (still using up the collagen)
- 3 raw egg yolks
- 12 oz steak
- 1 scrambled egg
- 2 oz cheese
- Buttered decaf coffee

Day 20

I am continuing to have zero cravings for anything – though I do find that I enjoy buttered coffee more than ever. I am making sourdough bread for my family and I do not have any desire for it. Strange.

I still have matcha tea, jasmine green tea, and coffee. I will slowly use up those items in my kitchen, and then make decisions on whether to eliminate altogether.

We are going to be traveling the world and I can't see eating this way forever. I do see it as a good choice for extended periods if that's all I can manage due to travel and costs of meat abroad.

I feel great. I sleep well. I wake ready to wake. My skin is soft and glowy. So far, I have zero complaints on zero carb carnivore. (Note: eggs and cheese have a tiny amount of carb.)

- Matcha green tea
- Buttered collagen coffee
- Scrambled eggs
- 2 oz cheese
- 4 smoked oysters
- Mint tea
- 2 beef patties with cheese

Day 21

Today I continue feeling great. Went to the doc for women's wellness exam. My weight was great at 121 pounds and my blood pressure was 108/70.

- Black coffee
- Jasmine green tea
- 2 scrambled eggs
- Buttered collagen coffee
- Baked fish: cod

- Beef patties with cheese
- 1 egg and 2 oz cheese
- Rooibos tea

Day 22

I can go so long between meals eating a carnivore diet, whereas I previously used to think about my next meal soon after eating food with carbs. Update: Well I went for some cheese at 3pm because although I wasn't really hungry I just felt a bit weak. I'm probably still not eating enough on some days. I crashed with a two hour nap earlier as I had woken at 5am (went to bed at 10pm so that's not bad).

Thinking more… I also needed to get out of the condo. Get some fresh air. And with the large to-do list I keep chipping away at maybe my brain told me to nap.

- Black coffee
- 2 rooibos tea
- Buttered coffee with collagen
- 4 strips bacon
- 1/2 can wild caught sockeye salmon
- Buttered coffee
- 2 oz cheese
- Mint tea
- 2 beef and cheese patties

Day 23

Started my day waking well again. I had a small headache from dryness and sinuses, but it went away.

- Coffee
- Green jasmine tea
- Bacon
- Buttered collagen coffee
- Steak
- Coffee (though not really in the mood for it)
- Steak

Day 24

Feeling great still.

- Eggs cooked in ghee
- Buttered collagen coffee
- Beef patties with cheese and butter

- Green tea

Day 25
- Jasmine green tea
- 3-4 oz steak
- 20 oz buttered collagen coffee (have to be out and about for the day and this will keep me fueled a bit)
- 3 oz steak
- 3 oz beef patty with cheese
- 3 beef/pork brats! YUM!

Day 26

I can't get over how great my skin looks. I'm a believer that skin health comes from the inside and I've heard more than a few times about the turnaround in people's skin after going carnivore but… what were they eating before? I had a "clean and healthy" fat-rich omnivore diet prior to going carnivore, so I didn't have much to improve upon with my skin, or so I thought.

I love the evenness of my emotions and feeling of empowerment of not being a slave to food. I know that I can go long periods without food and I will be fine. This way of eating keeps me satiated for much longer than when I used to eat carbs. To be clear, it's not like my life sucked before eating a carnivore diet, it's just that I'm experiencing improvements I didn't expect.

- 5 eggs cooked with bacon fat and topped with butter
- Buttered coffee with collagen
- Rooibos tea
- Mint tea
- 4 pork/beef brats
- Oysters/sardines
- 2 oz cheese
- 2 brats

Day 27
- Tea
- Coffee
- Buttered collagen coffee
- 2-3 eggs in extra ghee
- 2 brats
- 1 oz cheese

- bits of tuna
- Buttered coffee
- 2 big beef patties with cheese

Day 28

Still feeling very well. Everything is as it has been lately, with easy food prep, feeling well, etc. I will say that today I ate more in the meat department. I was able to consume more than usual before I felt really full. Maybe that's because I'm getting used to this, as I have heard people don't start out eating a lot and have to "eat meat like it's their job" to help ensure success. I feel like I've graduated. I also noted today that, like, wow, I haven't had any carbs in almost a month which means no sugar. I've never done that!

- Tea
- Coffee
- Buttered collagen coffee
- 3.5 brats
- 1-2 oz cheese
- 2.5 patties with cheese

Day 29

I like how easy this eating style is. I feel free even in social situations because really you can find meat anywhere, might not always be the best kind, but it is available.

Today I added some coconut oil and MCT oil to my buttered coffee, making it "Bulletproof" because I have a small vial left of the mixture and thought I'd experiment to see what happens. No desire or need to buy those things anymore, but I had it on hand and thought I'd try.

Update: Yes, it bothered my stomach either the coconut oil, the MCT, or both maybe.

- Black coffee
- "Bulletproof Coffee" (butter, coconut oil, MCT, collagen powder)
- 14 oz steak
- 4 pork/beef spicy brats
- 4 smoked oysters
- 1/2 can sockeye salmon (canned)
- Black coffee

Day 30

I'm not going to stop even though this is day 30. We leave for Denmark in the beginning of March, and my plan is to stick with this at least until then. Steaks and patties and beef sound better to me than they did even in the first couple of weeks of eating this way. I'm able to take in a bit more meat, too. Woke up with a small sinus headache, nasal passages feel dry.

- Black coffee
- Buttered collagen coffee (still using up the collagen and then I won't buy again)
- 2 beef patties with cheese
- 2 sardines

Day 31

OM-GOODNESS I went 30 days as of last night as a carnivore. I think the butter helps me increase the fat in my diet when my meats aren't fatty enough. I wonder how nasty buttered hot water would be? I remember Dave Asprey making a delicious recipe of hot buttered water with stevia and vanilla added. It was damn tasty. But, plain buttered water? Yuck is my guess. What if I salted it? Hmmm … Hot Salted Butter Water? Ha, maybe not.

I had a minimal appetite for the first 10-14 days then it gradually increased as I "ate meat like it was my job." This helped to ensure nutrition and energy. I felt very good most of the days except for small headache and energy dips the first few days. Small sinus headache still today (started yesterday).

No bloat. Ever. Body composition is great. Always a flat stomach. Firm and taut.

Muscles in my arms look great.

- 2 cups black coffee
- 3 eggs scrambled in ghee
- Buttered coffee (small amount of butter)
- Steak

Day 32

Still finishing off headache so started the day with coffee. I feel like I could've done without the buttered coffee tonight and the extra cheese, but we had a weird day and my schedule got the better of me.

- Coffee x 2
- Matcha (had a more nervous morning and matcha calms me)
- 4 brats
- Chunk of cheese (1-2 oz)
- Chunk of cheese (1-2 oz)
- 2 beef patties with cheese slice on each
- Buttered coffee

Day 33

- Coffee

- Jasmine green tea
- 2 eggs scrambled in ghee
- Buttered collagen coffee
- Matcha
- Chipotle restaurant: I call it my "carnivore" bowl: 1 serving chicken: 3 servings steak (probably ate 3/4 of it)
- coffee
- 1 oz cheese
- 3 beef patties, broiled, no cheese

Day 34

Woke after 7 hours of sleep, like clockwork. Wanted coffee which was great, but I question my desire for it. I'd rather wake ambivalent. Going to have a couple of days of ribeyes and see how it goes. My goodness I drank a lot of decaf today.

- Coffee
- Buttered coffee
- 1/2 can salmon
- 3-4 slices bacon
- Ribeye
- Decaf
- 2 x iced decaf

Day 35

- Coffee
- Decaf
- Jasmine green tea
- Ribeye
- Perrier sparkling mineral water + heavy splash of whipping cream (I didn't care for this)
- Ribeye

Day 36

Yep, I'm having coffee. Today we leave for NY and the United Nations, so it's a day of travel. So much for giving it up. (Shameless plug: My husband co-authored a fantastic book series — STEAMTeam 5 — aimed at getting more girls into science and technology. That's why he was invited to speak at the U.N.)

- Large coffee with butter and collagen protein powder

- Beef sticks (like jerky)
- Venison jerky (ick, not good)
- Ribeye

(Here, for brevity, I skip a few repetitive days of my journal.)

Day 40
- Coffee
- Decaf
- Ribeye
- Ribeye
- Cheese

Day 41
- Coffee
- Buttered collagen decaf
- Ribeye
- Ribeye

Day 42
Didn't feel super after the cappuccino with heavy cream listed below. Maybe dairy isn't my friend anymore? Or maybe I just had too much.
- Coffee
- 4 strips bacon
- 1/2 can tuna
- 5 pieces salami
- 1 slice cheese
- 2 strips bacon
- 1/2 can tuna
- San Pellegrino sparkling mineral water
- Ground beef with mustard butter sauce
- Decaf cappuccino with heavy cream
- Decaf with heavy cream

Day 43
- Black coffee
- Green tea
- Buttered decaf

- 3 sardines and 8 smoked oysters
- 10 slices salami 2 oz cheese
- 3 eggs (felt nauseous after)
- Ground beef and butter with mustard

Day 44

I'm still trying to get my head around how much I should be eating and it's been over a month. I feel like I could scale back the amount I'm eating. I worked out today – definitely stronger than the last time I worked out a few months ago.

- Coffee
- Green tea
- Buttered coffee
- 4 pieces bacon
- 3 raw egg yolks
- Buttered decaf
- 1 oz raw cheese
- 1+ lb ribeye
- 8 oz coffee 1/2 reg 1/2 decaf
- Decaf with heavy cream
- T-bone steak cooked on the grill (I hadn't planned on eating again, but my brother was in town and he cooked steaks on the grill)

Day 45

- Decaf coffee
- Americano (dammit I just love coffee)
- Green tea
- Buttered decaf (before working out so I had at least a bit of fuel)
- Leftover T-bone steak (post workout fuel)
- Buttered decaf
- T-bone lunch
- 4 pork/beef brats dinner

And Then I Stopped Eating Carnivore… Temporarily

I ended up going about 70 days on the carnivore diet before I had to stop. I stopped only because we left the U.S. to travel around Europe for a while. Beef was expensive, I started eating less of it. I ate more eggs and dairy, canned mackerel, and occasional plant-based foods.

Both my husband's muscle mass and mine suffered from the lower protein (and maybe it's from the lack of beef specifically). Consistent resistance training is a challenge when you travel.

We had noticed that our atrophy from not working out slowed down when we were on high protein diets. We had never experienced this before; it felt almost magical... stop working out but don't lose mass? Or at least, not quickly? Amazing.

But when the protein levels dropped, so did the muscle mass, which was a bit disheartening.

But then, I found reliable sources for low-cost meat! (Tesco in UK, Aldi in France.) Once again, I was eating strictly carnivore, and mostly beef!

The forced hiatus and re-starting proved to be an interesting accidental experiment. In almost no time at all, my muscle tone started to return (despite doing only minimal maintenance-type workouts, using body-weight exercises since I had no access to a gym). Just like the first time I was strict carnivore, I found it shockingly easy to maintain my physique.

It's still too early to say how things will go longer term, such as six months, a year, or even more, but for now, it feels a bit like I've hit on a secret formula for low-workout-intensity muscle maintenance. And all of the other benefits described earlier above (clear skin, good sleep, less joint pain, etc.) — these too got a bit worse when I went off carnivore, and then quickly got better again when I started eating only meat.

My primary foods currently are:

- Ground beef (daily)
- Chicken drumsticks (every 2 to 3 days)

My occasional foods are:

- Canned mackerel (every 3 to 4 days)
- High-fat dairy (every 5 to 7 days)
- Eggs (every 2 to 4 days, unless it's in the meat)
- Cured meats (every 5 to 7 days)

CPSIA information can be obtained
at www.ICGtesting.com
Printed in the USA
LVHW101100300721
693916LV00007B/555